Recent Advances in Depression

Other Titles of Interest

KAHN, J. and EARLE, E.
The Cry For Help: and the Professional Response

LYNN, R.
Dimensions of Personality

MANGAN, G. L.
The Biology of Human Conduct

MILLER, W. R.
The Addictive Behaviors

RACHMAN, S.
Contributions to Medical Psychology, Volumes 1 & 2

Recent Advances in Depression

Edited by
C. N. STEFANIS

PERGAMON PRESS

OXFORD · NEW YORK · TORONTO · SYDNEY · PARIS · FRANKFURT

U.K.	Pergamon Press Ltd., Headington Hill Hall, Oxford OX3 0BW, England
U.S.A.	Pergamon Press Inc., Maxwell House, Fairview Park, Elmsford, New York 10523, U.S.A.
CANADA	Pergamon Press Canada Ltd., Suite 104, 150 Consumers Rd., Willowdale, Ontario M2J 1P9, Canada
AUSTRALIA	Pergamon Press (Aust.) Pty. Ltd., P.O. Box 544, Potts Point, N.S.W. 2011, Australia
FRANCE	Pergamon Press SARL, 24 rue des Ecoles, 75240 Paris, Cedex 05, France
FEDERAL REPUBLIC OF GERMANY	Pergamon Press GmbH, Hammerweg 6, D – 6242 Kronberg-Taunus, Federal Republic of Germany

Copyright © 1983 Pergamon Press Ltd.

All Rights Reserved. No part of this publication may be reproduced, stored in a retrieval system or transmitted in any form or by any means: electronic, electrostatic, magnetic tape, mechanical, photocopying, recording or otherwise, without permission in writing from the publishers.

First edition 1983

Library of Congress Cataloging in Publication Data

Main entry under title:
Recent advances in depression.
1. Depression, Mental. I. Stefanis, C. N. [DNLM:
1. Depression—Congresses. WM 171 R295 1980]
RC537.R4   1982   616.85'27   82-18556

British Library Cataloguing in Publication Data

Recent advances in depression.
1. Depression, Mental — Congresses
I. Stefanis, C.N.
616.85'27   RC537
ISBN 0-08-027954-6

In order to make this volume available as economically and as rapidly as possible the authors' typescripts have been reproduced in their original forms. This method unfortunately has its typographical limitations but it is hoped that they in no way distract the reader.

Printed in Great Britain by A. Wheaton & Co. Ltd., Exeter

Contents

Introductory Remarks   vii
C. N. Stefanis

1. Genetic Aspects of Depression

1. Genetics of depressive disorders   1
   J. Mendlewicz
2. Affective disorders and ABO blood types: A critical review   13
   P. Rinieris and C. Stefanis
3. Comparative investigation of two pairs of monozygotic twins, one with and the other without endogenous depression   17
   B. Alevizos et al.

2. Clinical Aspects of Depression

1. Psychopathology of depression   27
   K. Achté
2. Hostility in depression   35
   G. C. Lyketsos
3. The role of aggression in affective disorders and its relationship to anxiety   41
   A. Liakos et al.
4. The relation of obsessive-compulsive phenomena to anxiety in depressive patients   49
   J. Liappas, A. D. Rabavilas and C. Stefanis
5. Depression in the institutionalized elderly   53
   C. Soldatos

3. Psychological and Epidemiological Aspects of Depression

1. Psychometric aspects of the depressions   59
   M. Hamilton
2. Depressive symptoms in a Greek population sample: investigation with the MMPI   65
   A. Kokkevi et al.
3. Sex differences in depression: observations on an outpatient psychiatric sample   73
   M. Markidis et al.
4. Masked depression and immigration   79
   M. G. Madianos

4. Biological Aspects of Depression

1. Recent advances in the biology of depression   87
   W. E. Bunney Jr. and B. L. Garland

2. Cellular factors in manic depressive illness: blood and brain 99
   M. R. Issidorides
3. Clinical and biological correlates of a 48-hour cycling manic- 109
   depressive patient
   G. Trikkas et al.
4. Neuroendocrine derangements in depression 117
   G. Tolis
5. Thyrotropin and prolactin responses to thyrotropin-releasing 129
   hormone stimulation test in male inpatients with psychotic and
   neurotic depression
   A. Martinos et al.

5. Treatment Aspects of Depression

1. Current treatment for depression 133
   P. Kielholz
2. The risks and adverse effects of ECT 143
   R. E. Kendell
3. Psychometric, electroencephalographic and histochemical 151
   changes following long-term lithium administration. Preliminary
   observations
   G. N. Christodoulou et al.
4. Sleep deprivation in the prophylaxis of manic-depressive illness 157
   G. N. Christodoulou et al.

Introductory Remarks

C. N. Stefanis

Department of Psychiatry, Athens University Medical School, Athens, Greece

Depression as a diagnostic term appeared in the Psychiatric Literature only recently, early in this century. No one has claimed fame for coining it and no one can feel justified for having adopted it. Having been widely used over the years to designate not only a particular mental disorder but also all the varieties of emotional reactions to actual or anticipated loss, depression has lost its initial semantic value. Severe affective psychopathology is frequently confused with feelings of sorrow and distress arising from adverse life events.

It is thus no wonder, as recent studies have shown, that the average individual views depression as part of life experience, an unavoidable condition that every one has to go through at least once in his life-time and considers it subject to self-cure by will power. Needless to say that this kind of attitude by failing to distinguish between transient dysphoric loss-related emotional states and clinical depression leading to profound disturbance of mental and social functioning is both unrealistic and hazardous. In contrast to the normal emotional responses to unwanted and stressful events clinical depression is a mental disorder, which due to its severity, its tendency to recur and its high cost for the individual and the society,constitutes one of today's major public health problems.

It is estimated that more than 150 milion people in the world present symptoms of clinical depression. Suicide, manifesting the self-destructive aspect of this disorder, ranks as second or third leading cause of death among the young (15-24 years of age). More than a thousand people commit suicide every day and in Europe only more than 100.000 deaths per year are officially registered as due to suicide. Considering the under-reporting, the great number of suicidal attempts with narrow escape due to chance factors and to early and life-saving interventions, one may have a measure of the magnitude of the suicide problem that is so closely related to depression.

Moreover, as we all know, the feeling state and the behavioural manifestations of the depressed individual,contribute substantially to family disorganization, job loss, early retirement, alcoholism, drug dependence and traffic accidents.

Finally, regarding the social cost, we have only to refer to results from recent surveys which indicate that over one third of patients contacting General Health Services and being subjected to unnecessary expensive medical examinations,have psychiatric problems,usually depression masked in physical symptoms.

Depression appears in various clinical forms and the accumulated data over the years indicate that not only the symptomatology and severity,but also the clinical course,as well as the etiological factors,differ in the two major diagnostic groups of depression: the endogenous or psychotic or primary and the neurotic or reactive or secondary. It is mainly the former group that received attention and has become the center of research efforts in the past few years. This is due, in part, to the recognition of biological and genetic factors associated with "endogenous" depression and certainly to the realization that this type of affective illness is the most serious in terms of personal suffering and social cost.

The progressively increasing flow of information in the past few years on all the aspects of this diagnostic group of depression, witnesses to the fact that research in this area has been fruitful and most rewarding. Findings derived from twin, adoption and family studies, in conjunction with the search for biological markers, have convincingly demonstrated the involvement of genetic factors to their etiology and have also substantially contributed to their diagnostic subtyping. Animal experiments and clinical neuropharmacology studies on the mode of action of antidepressant drugs, together with neurochemical investigation of body fluids from patients during and after depressive or manic episodes, revealed a link between psychopathology of the affective illness and changes in the activity of the central aminergic synaptic system: In fact the monoamine hypothesis formulated on the basis of these studies, dominated the field for the past two decades and has determined the course of pharmaceutical research for the development of new antidepressant agents. Chronobiological studies, in association with clinical and EEG sleep studies, have demonstrated in depressed patients specific changes in diurnal biorhythmicity and provided us with a deeper insight in to the psychophysiology of depression. Furthermore, the increasing interest in psychoneuroendocrinology has led to the more recent exciting discoveries of the close association that exists between affective illness and dysfunction of the hypothalamic retino-pineal and possibly of higher brain centers governing hormonal secretion. The implications of these discoveries may prove to be far greater than currently recognized. By the time that this book will be published we anticipate that more data will appear that may provide clinical psychiatry with a useful laboratory tool to facilitate diagnostic procedure, follow up, and prediction of treatment response.

It is though to be realized that what has been achieved so far, has only paved the way that will eventually lead to unravelling the enigma of affective illness. We still do not fully understand why and how an individual falls into depression. We still have data which do not fit together and other which cannot be integrated into a single conceptual framework. Findings are plenty, but sound knowledge is still ahead of us.

In order to accelerate progress, it is urgent to improve communication between researchers in the field. Priority should be given to the establishment of a classification system for affective disorders with universally accepted strict diagnostic criteria. All the existing systems should be integrated by WHO Expert Committees into a single comprehensive system that will enable researchers around the world to speak the same scientific language and acquire a common frame of reference.

A major portion of the classification problem is the clarification of terms. Terms to be used, should semantically differentiate between types of depression. As already mentioned the term depression may not adequately serve this purpose. If to be retained, it should be preferably used to denote a symptom rather than a nosological entity. The term melancholia instead may be the most appropriate to designate those affective disorders that are presently known as endogenous, primary, major and psychotic. Hippocrates may have failed to recognize mania and melancholia as the two dipoles of the same disease process, but what he described it fully corresponds to the basic clinical features of the affective illness that all of the above terms intend to signify.

Lastly, efforts at an international level for a more integrated approach to the problem of affective disorders should be encouraged. Opportunities for researchers from the Clinic and from the Laboratory to exchange findings and views should be increased in order to attain a unified concept on the identity of these disorders. The present Symposium attempted to meet such a need.

Introductory Remarks

The meeting was organized by the Department of Psychiatry of Athens University (Eginition Hospital) and aimed at reviewing recent advances and indentifying the critical areas in which future research on affective disorders will have to be directed. Scientists of a world-wide reputation for their research work have authoritatively reviewed developments in their respective field of interest and presented original findings of their current work. Within the framework of these informative papers, the findings from a number of studies in the area of affective disorders which were carried out by various research groups in our Department, have been reported and jointly discussed.

The Proceedings of the meeting which include data from ongoing research and comphrehensive reviews, may hopefully provide the reader with material informative on the current state of knowledge in the field and useful for future research strategies.

COSTAS STEFANIS, M.D.
Professor and Chairman
Dept. of Psychiatry
University of Athens,
Eginition Hospital

1. Genetic Aspects of Depression

Genetics of Depressive Disorders

J. Mendlewicz

Department of Psychiatry, University of Brussels, School of Medicine, Brussels, Belgium

ABSTRACT

In the first section of this paper, a critical review of the epidemiological and genetic studies related to the affective disorders, is presented. Emphasis was placed on the existing evidence on the genetic distinction between bipolar and unipolar forms of affective disorders, as well as on the X-linked dominant factor involved in the transmission of the bipolar phenotype in at least some families. With regard to the mode of inheritance of bipolar illness, only three genetic models, i.e. that of a major autosomal dominant gene and that of a polygenic inheritance, seem to fit the genetic data published so far.
dels, i.e. that of a major autosomal dominant gene with reduced penetrance, that of an X-linked dominant gene and that of a polygenic inheritance, seem to fit the genetic data published so far.
In the second section of this paper, a review of the data on the relationships between affective disorders and schizophrenia, is presented. The evidence suggests that these major psychoses are genetically different and that the syndrome defined as schizo-affective illness still remains a puzzling problem, with regard to both clinical and genetic aspects.
In the third section of this paper, the problems at issue in the area of the genetics and nosology of schizophrenia, as well as the solutions to selected problems and their relevance to genetic councelling, are reviewed and discussed.

KEYWORDS

Epidemiology and heredity of affective disorders; relationships between affective disorders and schizophrenia; genetics and nosology of schizophrenia.

AFFECTIVE DISORDERS: EPIDEMIOLOGY AND HEREDITY.

Some investigators have recently discriminated between bipolar (manic-depressive) and unipolar (depressive) illness in affective disorder research (Leonhard, 1959). Bipolar patients experience both mania and depression, whereas unipolar patients experience depression only. Most of the epidemiological studies on affective disorders have not made this distinction and various investigators have used different diagnostic criteria for classifying the affective psychoses. It is therefore difficult to assess reliably the prevalence of affective illness in the general population. Several investigators, however, have reported lifetime risks for bipolar (manic-depressive) illness in various geographical areas under specific conditions. The rates published vary from a low of 0.07% (Böök, 1953) to a high of 7.0 (Tomasson, 1938).

The unusually low rate of 0.07% corresponds to only two cases of manic-depressive illness in a population of about 9.000 persons in a province of northern Sweden. Zerbin-Rüdin (1967), who reviewed most population studies in manic-depressive illness, places the overall rate for this disease at around 1%. This rate is consistent with, although not identical to, the rates published by Slater (1953) for Great Britain (0.5-0.8%), Sjögren (1948) for Sweden (0.6-0.8%), and Kallmann (1954) for New York State (0.4%). These differences in the prevalence of manic-depressive illness according to the country investigated could be partially explained by genetic factors: e.g., breeding effects and higher consanguinity rates in isolates in Scandinavia, or differences in ethnic backgrounds. However, environmental factors may also lead to such differences. Among these are sampling artifacts such as the different sizes of the samples studied, and the differences in the ethnic and socioeconomic composition of the populations investigated. Furthermore, some studies are based on admission to state hospitals and represent an incidence rate rather than a true prevalence, admissions to private and community facilities are rarely included in these surveys. This represents a serious bias since we know that population rates for a disease may fluctuate with time according to hospitalization policy or availability of beds. To illustrate this, the lifetime hospital admission risk for all affective disorders published by the Registrar General and the Ministry of Health in England in 1964 was 2.4% for males and 5.8% for females, a nearly 50% rise for both sexes. These apparently low or high rates in certain areas may be true only under special demographic conditions. In addition to differences in sampling, investigators utilize different statistical procedures and, more important, various diagnostic criteria. American psychiatrists tend to diagnose schizophrenia more frequently and underdiagnose manic-depressive illness as compared to their British and Western European colleagues who are more prone to diagnose affective illness (Cooper and co-workers, 1972). Nevertheless, one may conclude from the more reliable lifetime risk studies that 1 % would be a conservative rate for the prevalence of bipolar manic-depressive illness in the general population (Ministry of Health, London, 1969). If one were to include milder forms of bipolar illness and unipolar illness, where a considerable number of subjects are being treated as outpatients, the general prevalence may well be as high as 10 %.

Most studies have reported an appreciable difference between the sexes in the distribution of manic-depressive illness (Helgasson, 1964). The sexes ratio generally accepted is two females to one male. The interpretation of this excess of females is still controversial. It is conceivable that for cultural reasons, women are more likely to be hospitalized for manic-depressive illness than men. If this were true, one would expect to find the same phenomenon for schizophrenia, something that remains to be proved. Another possible explanation is the fact that male suicides outnumber female suicides by ratio of about 2 to 1 (Rüdin, 1923). Finally, one could also invoke the hypothesis of sex-limited factors, e.g., hormonal (Zerbin-Rübin, 1967) or sex-linked genetic factors, increasing the expressivity of manic-depressive illness in females predisposed to this disorder.

The twin method allows comparison of concordance rates for a trait between sets of monozygotic (MZ) and dizygotic (DZ) twins. Both types of twins share a similar environement, but they are genetically different. Monozygotic twins behave genetically as identical individuals, whereas DZ twins share only half of their genes and thus behave as sibs. Most twin studies show that the concordance rate for manic-depressive illness in MZ twins is significantly higher than the concordance rate for the disease in DZ twins (Zerbin-Rübin, 1969). This observation is taken as evidence in favor of a genetic factor in manic-depressive illness.

Table 1 gives the concordance rate for affective disorder in MZ and DZ twins,according to various investigators who reported on 20 or more pairs(Rosanoff and co-workers, 1934; Da Fonseca, 1959; Harvald and Hauge, 1965; Kringlen, 1967). The concordance rates in MZ twins vary between 50 and 92.5 % (mean 69.3 %) as compared to 0-38.5 % in DZ twins (mean 20 %). These results strongly support the presence of a genetic factor in the etiology of manic-depressive illness.

TABLE 1 Concordance rates for manic-depressive illness in twins

Ref.	Concordance rate (%)	
	MZ	DZ
Rosanoff and co-workers (1934)	69.6	16.4
Kallman (1954)	92.6	23.6
Da Fonseca (1959)	71.4	38.5
Harvald and Hauge (1965)	50.0	2.6
Kringlen (1967)	33.3	0.0

Price reviewed the twin literature in order to locate pairs of identical twins who had been reared apart since early childhood and who were characterized by at least one of the twins being diagnosed as affectively ill (Price, 1968). Price was able to find 12 such pairs of MZ twins. Among these pairs, eight were concordant for the disease, an observation suggesting that the predisposition to manic-depressive illness will usually express itself regardless of the early environment. The complex interaction between hereditary and environmental factors underlying the etiology of manic-depressive illness cannot be elucidated by the twin method, nor can it tell us the type of genetic mechanisms that may be involved in the transmission of manic-depressive illness.
Most of the early studies on manic-depressive illness have shown that this illness tends to be familial (Kallmann, 1954). The lifetime risk for the disease in relatives of manic-depressive probands is significantly higher than the risk in the general population. The risks published by Kallmann (1954) for parents of manic-depressive probands is 23.4% and for sibs 22.7%. With regard to morbidity risks in the more distant relatives (second-degree relatives), the rates usually range from 1 to 4%. It is thus clear that the risks for the illness are decreased as the degree of consanguinity is lowered, as expected if there is a genetic component in the etiology of this disease.
Most of the early family studies have been influenced by Kraepelin's classification as far as nosology is conserned. As a result of this, the aforementioned investigators have included among their probands patients suffering from mania and depression (bipolar) and patients presenting depression only (unipolar) without distinguishing between these. Thus, the samples investigated in the various studies are relatively heterogeneous. Leonhard (1959) in Berlin was one of the first investigators to make a clinical distinction between bipolar and unipolar forms of affective disorders on genetic grounds. The bipolar patients were shown to have a greater genetic loading for affective disorder than the unipolar patients. They also had more relatives with hypomanic temperaments as compared to the unipolar patients, whose relatives had depressive temperaments. It was concluded that bipolar and unipolar disorders may have different genetic etiologies. Two recent independent studies have investigated bipolar and unipolar probands separately (Angst, 1966; Perris, 1968). Both studies found that the morbidity risks for affective disorders were significantly higher in the relatives of bipolar as compared to unipolar patients. Bipolar and unipolar illnesses were present in the relatives of bipolar patients, whereas only unipolar illness was found in the relatives of unipolar patients. This genetic distinction between unipolar and bipolar illness has recently been confirmed by Winokur and co-workers (1969) in the United States. In this study the lifetime risks for affective illness (i.e., bipolar and unipolar) in the first-degree relatives of bipolar patients were 34% for parents and 35% for sibs. These rates are similar to those we have found in studying the relatives of 134 bipolar probands in New York City (Mendlewicz and Rainer, 1974) Table 2 illustrates age-corrected risks found in various types of first-degree relatives of bipolar patients. This table indicates that the type of affective disorder found in the relatives of bipolar patients is not restricted to bipolar illness. The risk for unipolar illness is indeed quite significant in these relatives. The overall rates for affectives illness are similar in sibs and parents; however, sibs are

more likely to manifest bipolar illness than parents.

TABLE 2 Morbidity risks for affective illness in relatives
of bipolar manic-depressive patients
(a,b)

	All affective %	Bipolar %	Unipolar %
Parents	33.7±2.9	12.1±2.0	22.0±2.6
Sibs	39.2±3.0	21.2±2.5	18.6±2.5
Children	59.9±6.0	24.6±5.0	41.3±6.7

a From Mendlewicz and Rainer (1974)
b N=134

It can be seen that children of bipolar probands constitute a high-risk group. After reviewing all family studies, the risk for manic-depressive illness in the relatives of affected patients can be estimated at somewhere between 15 and 35%. There is, however, a large proportion of relatives of bipolar probands who exhibit unipolar illness only. When correction has been made for age, diagnoses, and statistical procedures, the morbidity risks for manic-depressive illness in different types of first-degree relatives (parents, sibs, children) are similar. This observation is consistent with a dominant mode of transmission in this disease.

A number of studies have reported that the O blood group is most frequently found in manic-depressive patients (Parker and co-workers, 1961; Mendlewicz and co-workers, 1974). This potential association between a blood group factor and a major psychosis, although poorly understood, may indicate that the ABO genotype plays a role in the predisposition to manic-depressive illness. Association between traits is not to be confused with linkage, i.e., the proximity of two traits on the same chromosome resulting in their dependent assortment during the process of meiosis. In this type of study, one tries to test a potential linkage relationship between a known genetic marker and a character known to be genetically determined, but which has not yet been mapped on the chromosomes. This method has been used successfully in the genetic study of several hereditary conditions (Renwick and Schulze, 1964; Fialkow and co-workers, 1967), and has recently been used to test the hypothesis of X linkage in manic-depressive illness.

Reich and co-workers (1969) studied two large families assorting for color blindness (an X-linked recessive marker) and manic-depressive illness. Mendlewicz and co-workers (1972a) reported on seven such families. In both studies the marker and the illness failed to show independent assortment. Winokur and Tanna (1969) described three more families assorting in a dependent fashion for manic-depressive illness and the Xg blood group (a dominant X-linked marker). We have confirmed these results in 11 other families assorting for the Xg blood group and the illness (Mendlewicz and co-workers, in press). In a more recent study, Mendlewicz and Fleiss (1974) were able to demonstrate close linkage between bipolar illness and both deutan* and protan* color blindness in 17 informative pedigrees.

---

*Deutan color blindness is a deficiency of green perception; protan is a deficiency of red perception. The chromosomal loci of these two conditions are closely linked but not identical.

Linkage between bipolar illness and the Xg blood group, although measurable, was found to be less close in 23 informative families. These linkage results, originating from different laboratories, suggest that an X-linked dominant factor is involved in the transmission of the manic-depressive phenotype in at least some families. The findings of close linkage between bipolar illness and the color vision loci, and of less close linkage between the illness and the Xg blood group have to be interpreted in the light of the fact that the loci for the Xg blood group and color-blindness seem to be far apart. Thus, the locus for bipolar illness appears to be between the Xg locus and the color-blindness loci, probably closer to the latter. However, we were unable to measure linkage between unipolar depressive illness and either protanopia or the Xg blood group, in 14 informative families (Mendlewicz and Fleiss, 1974), an observation ruling out X-linked inheritance as the mode of transmission of unipolar illness. These negative results for unipolar illness are important in the light of the positive findings concerning X linkage in bipolar families, because all families studied by us were obtained from the same sample during the same period. The linkage studies conducted so far on manic-depressive illness are of great value since they are able to discriminate between sex-linked and sex-influenced types of inheritance and they do provide an estimate of the significance of the results. They all point to the presence of an X-linked dominant factor in the transmission of manic-depressive illness. This methodological approach is of great potential and should be extended to the study of other psychiatric conditions such as schizophrenia, using other genetic markers located on different chromosomes.

A recent adoption study showing more psychopathology of the affective spectrum in biological parents of manic-depressive adoptees as compared to their adoptive parents is further evidence in favor of the genetic hypothesis of affective illness (Mendlewicz and Rainer, 1977).

There is no final consensus on the types of genetic mechanisms that operate in affective illness. Too little is known about the genetics of unipolar and schizoaffective illness to even propose specific genetic models for these syndromes in this chapter. It is even difficult, if not impossible, to draw definite conclusions on the mode of inheritance of bipolar manic-depressive illness. First, as we have said before, bias in selecting study populations must be carefully avoided, and second, clinical or genetic heterogeneity may foil the attempt to draw an unequivocal conclusion. There are, however, certain genetic models that can be ruled out from the genetic data published so far. Autosomal recessive inheritance is one of these, since it cannot account for the appreciable number of families showing a two- and three-generation transmission of the illness. There is no increase in morbid risks in sibs and consanguinity, which would be expected under recessive inheritance. Sex-linked recessive inheritance is also very unlikely because there are no studies so far reporting an excess of affected males over affected females. In fact, the opposite has generally been observed.

There are some arguments in favor of a major dominant type of inheritance (a). The illness has often been observed to be present in successive generations; (b) the morbidity risks in parents, sibs, and children are similar and some studies have shown the risks in sibs of probands with no affected parents to be equal to the risks in sibs with one affected parent (Stenstedt, 1952; Winokur and co-workers; 1969) and (c) when we tested our own data for consistency with a single-gene threshold model using a modification of a program developed by Kidd and Cavalli-Sforza (1973), the observed values for sibs and parents were compatible with various forms of single-gene inheritance, with dominant inheritance most likely (Mendlewicz and Rainer, 1974).

Single-factor inheritance is consistent with these data. Some investigators have postulated a major autosomal dominant gene with reduced penetrance for manic-depressive illness (Strömgren, 1938; Stenstedt, 1952; Kallmann, 1954). This autosomal hypothesis has the value of simplicity and fits most of the data except for the sex ratio differences found in patients and relatives, i.e., a preponderance of affected females. Polygenic inheritance in bipolar manic-depressive illness has

also been suggested by other investigators who used a computational model to test
ancestral secondary cases for polygenic versus monogenic inheritance (Perris, 1972;
Slater and co-workers, 1972). However, another study using the same method has
shown that one subgroup of the illness conformed to a monogenic model while a second subgroup behaved as a polygenic entity (Mendlewicz and co-workers, 1973).
Finally, the linkage studies described in the preceding section contribute strong
evidence which points to an X-linked dominant gene involved in the transmission of
some manic-depressive illness. A more recent family study arrives at the same conclusion for early onset forms of bipolar illness (Taylor and Abrams, 1974). It is
argued, however, that there are families where male-to-male transmission of the
disease is apparent, an observation incompatible with X-linkage (Perris, 1968;
Goetzl and co-workers, 1974). This is also the case in our own material (Mendlewicz and Rainer, 1974), where these families represent about 10% of our overall
sample. Furthermore, the preponderance of affected females as compared to males in
first-degree relatives (Angst, 1966; Winokur and co-workers, 1969; Mendlewicz and
Rainer, 1974; Taylor and Abrams, 1974) of bipolar patients is far from a universal
finding (Perris, 1968; Brown and co-workers, 1973; Goetzl and co-workers, 1974).
An interesting approach to the problem has recently been proposed by Crowe and
Smouse (1974). These authors, working on Winokur's data, have derived an age-dependent penetrance function for manic-depressive illness. Their analysis revealed
that a sex-linked dominant model was far more likely to explain the data than an
autosomal dominant one. Although we are suggesting that the X-linked dominant model is the preponderant mode of transmission of manic-depressive illness, it seems
quite clear that more than one genetic entity is involved in this disease.

AFFECTIVE DISORDERS AND SCHIZOPHRENIA: GENETICS AND NOSOLOGY

There are few investigators who believe that schizophrenia and affective illness
are genetically related. Most genetic studies have concluded that these two major
psychoses are genetically different. The morbidity risks for schizophrenia in first-degree relatives (except for children) of manic-depressive probands are the same as in the general population (Angst, 1966; Zerbin-Rüdin, 1967; Perris, 1968;
Winokur and co-workers, 1969). There is, however, one exception to this rule: involutional melancholia. Kallman (1954) has reported the risks for schizophrenia to
 be three to four times higher in the relatives of involutional patients than in
the general population.
This finding is rather surprising since involutional disease is of late onset and
schizophrenia usually starts early in life. The risk for schizophrenia in children of bipolar manic-depressive parents has also been found to be slightly elevated (∿ 3%) (kallmann, 1954). On the other hand, the risk for manic-depressive illness in the relatives of schizophrenia probands has generally been reported to be
low (Kallmann, 1954). Another argument in favor of a genetic distinction between
schizophrenia and affective illness is the absence of any reported instances of MZ
twins where one twin is schizophrenic and the other affectively ill. In Slater's
(1953) twin study, there is no single case of schizophrenia among the parents,
sibs, or cotwins of DZ twins diagnosed as affective disorder. There seems to be
little evidence, if any, favoring a genetic overlap between schizophrenia and affective illness. This does not mean that there is no overlap regarding the clinical manifestations of these illnesses. It is actually well documented that manic
patients experience schizophrenia-like symptoms (i.e., hallucinations, paranoid ideas, etc) and other atypical symptoms. These patients are often misdiagnosed as
schizophrenic, even though they present a recurrent type of disorder with full remissions between the episodes (Clayton and co-workers, 1968; Mendlewicz and co-workers, 1972b). We also know of schizophrenic patients suffering from a chronic condition who may experience mania or depression. At the present time, those disorders with mixed clinical symptomatology are often labeled "schizo-affective"; they
seem to have a complex and unclear relationship to either schizophrenia or affective illness. Schizo-affective illness is classified according to the American Psy-

chiatric Association nomenclature as a subgroup of schizophrenia, but we have to point out that so far there are no data to support this hypothesis. A natural inbreeding experiment can be found in the few studies describing matings between a schizophrenic and a manic-depressive parent (Smith, 1925; Schultz, 1940, Elsasser, 1952).
These studies have shown equal risks for schizophrenia and manic-depressive illness in the children. No children were diagnosed as schizo-affective, an observation indicating that the schizo-affective phenotype does not result from a combination of schizophrenic and manic genes. Some investigators have suggested that schizo-affective illness is genetically related to affective illness (Weiner and Strömgren, 1958; Clayton and co-workers, 1968; Abrams and co-workers, 1974).
Clayton and co-workers (1968) conducted family studies on 39 schizo-affective patients. They found a high prevalence of affective disorder in these families, while schizophrenia and schizo-affective pscyhosis was found to be rare in the relatives of their probands. On the basis of these results, they concluded that schizo-affective psychosis was just a variant of affective disorder. Asano (1967) in Japan, studying atypical cases of manic-depressive illness with schizophrenia-like symptoms, also found affective illness to be present in the relatives of the patients. The risks for affective illness in the relatives of atypical cases were, however, lower than in the relatives of typical manic-depressive patients.
In a large twin study on 15.909 veteran pairs, Cohen and co-workers (1972) reviewed the charts of 420 twin pairs where one or both twins had a psychotic diagnosis. The MZ pairwise concordance rate for schizo-affective illness was significantly higher than the one found for schizophrenia, and was much closer to the one found for manic-depressive illness. The similarity found in genotypic/phenotypic variance between manic-depressive and schizo-affective twins led these authors to conclude that there exist common genetic determinants for these two illnesses. It is conceivable that the pathogenesis of schizo-affective psychosis may include some genetic factor similar to that of manic-depressive psychosis, but its full expression may require the presence of personality and environmental factors in the origin of schizophrenia. The possibility can also be considered that schizo-affective disorder represents an autonomous entity distinct from schizophrenia or affective illness or that a subject presenting schizo-affective symptoms has in fact two separate disorders. The latter hypothesis would explain why it is common to find in these families a mixed set of manic-depressive and schizophrenic relatives (Weiner and Strömgren, 1958; Strömgren, 1965; Belmaker and Wyatt, 1974). We may admit the fact that being a schizophrenic does not necessarily confer immunity against becoming manic-depressive, although this "association" may be difficult to understand from psychodynamic point of view. Furthermore even conservatively estimating the prevalence of schizophrenia and manic-depressive illness in the general population (∼1%), the probability of one individual to carry both diseases would be about 1 out of 10.000, a rather rare event.
We have reasons to believe that schizophrenia and manic-depressive illness represent two distinct genetic illnesses. The syndrome defined as schizo-affective illness still remains a puzzling problem, with regard to both clinical and genetic aspects; it deserves further investigation of its long-term clinical course and heredity.

SCHIZOPHRENIA: GENETICS AND NOSOLOGY.

Family risk studies, twin surveys, the model of adoption, and longitudinal investigations of high-risk children have been used successively to approach the numerous problems at issue in this area. These special problems are (a) diagnosis, (b) separation, at least in concept, of heredity and environment, (c) forms of inheritance and (d) developmental expression of genetic predisposition. In this section, an attempt is made to review some solutions to selected problems and indicate their relevance to genetic counseling.
Diagnosis has long been a concern of psychiatrists who want to understand the role

of heredity in mental disorder. They are often accused of making too few diagnostic distinctions in choosing their test populations, of making too many, or of using the wrong ones; of working with non homogeneous samples on the one hand, or with idiosyncratic or ad hoc divisions on the other; and of lacking clinical sensitivity to the individuality of human lives. Actually in the history of psychiatric genetics as a discipline, one of the main goals has been to clarify nosological distinctions and establish diagnosis on some kind of etiological basis. Thus, a genetic study may start with a broad selection of subjects, defined on symptomatic, social, or other pragmatic bases, and lead by a process of elimination to one or more clearly defined groups. This way seem a circular approach, but it is rather more like a spiral, leading to better defined and purer categories.
Until the identification of genetic, enzymatic, or metabolic errors makes it possible to identify the subclinical carrier, the genotype, or the "endophenotype" in schizophrenia, diagnosis has to be made on symptomatic grounds, on the basis of disease, or on the basis of structured interviews or psychological tests. Biological variables(nailfold capillary patterns, bodily constitution, chromosomal aneuploidy) has been implicated in some groups of schizophrenic patients, but none of them is pathognomonic.
However, genetics has made contributions to the problem of the nosology of schizophrenia in two levels. In the first place, it has addressed itself to the distinction between schizophrenia and other psychotic illnesses, particularly manic-depressive psychosis, and the correlation of schizophrenia with such syndromes as involutional psychosis. Lewis (1967) once wrote, "In the search for an essential identity underlying the difference between two psychiatric syndromes, the safest indication is a greater frequency of one of the syndromes in the families of propositi exhibiting the other syndrome than would be the case in families drawn at random from the general population". In Kallmann's (1946) twin family material, no twin pairs were found with both schizophrenia and manic-depressive psychosis, nor was there an increase in manic-depressive psychosis in family of schizophrenic twins or vice versa. Involutional psychosis was found more often than expected in the families of schizophrenics, and Kallmann felt that this diagnostic category was either less homogeneous clinically or more complex pathogenetically than either schizophrenia or manic-depressive psychosis.
In the second place, genetics has focused on the problems of heterogeneity within schizophrenia itself. In his first family study, Kallmann (1938) divided the cases into four types: the hebephrenic and the catatonic types, in which there was a degree of desintegration of personality, the paranoid type, and the simple type, which ran a mild course without any considerable deterioration. Among the offspring of these patients, he found that in the hebephrenic and catatonic types the expectancy rate for schizophrenia was about 21%, whereas in the paranoid and simple types it was about 11%. He was led by this finding to bracket the former two classes as the nuclear group and the latter two as the peripheral group. In sibs, the schizophrenia rate was about 13% in the nuclear group and about 9% in the peripheral group. Despite these consistent differences in expectancy, the four different disease forms did not correspond to different hereditary predispositions: The children of hebephrenic or paranoid patients were not always, in turn, hebephrenic or paranoid; and two or more patients in the same series of children did not manifest the same form of psychosis. Kallmann's conclusion was that the individual form of schizophrenia was determined by a series of subsidiary factors in addition to the main hereditary predisposition, and that the modifying factors might themselves be of a polygenic nature. Later, in his study of schizophrenic twins, Kallmann (1946) indicated a concordance rate as low as 26% for MZ cotwins of schizophrenic patients with little or no deterioration, with a range from 2 to 17% for DZ pairs. These findings were similar to the observations that were made in the series of Kringlen (1968) and Gottesman and Schields (1972), in which higher concordance rates were found among the cotwins of more seriously ill schizophrenic patients,. particularly of chronic patients.
In an early study by Shultz and Leonhard (1940) there were fewer cases of schizophrenia

in the parents of patients with typical than with atypical schizophrenia. There has recently been a tendency, on both clinical and genetic grounds, to divide schizophrenia into these two forms, one being known variously as the nuclear, endogenous, typical, process, or familial type and the other as the peripheral, exogenous, atypical, reactive, or schizophreniform type of schizophrenia. These categories overlap, and various investigators define them somewhat differently. The division into process and reactive forms, as described by Garmezy (1965) is based on the nature of the premorbid phase, the precipitating cause, and the prognosis or outcome. Process schizophrenia is preceded by a poorly integrated premorbid personality with inadequate behavior in many ways, social withdrawal, and no acute precipitants. The onset is an insidious one, with emotional blunting, apathy, and indifference, and long periods of secondary symptoms. Reactive schizophrenics, on the other hand, have shown generally good school and home adjustment, establishment of heterosexual and other friendly relationships, and then a precipitating event, overt expression of aggression and hostility, a fulminating course, many secondary symptoms, and good response to treatment.
In the typical-atypical dichotomy according to Langfeldt (1939), the typical form includes a prepsychotic schizoid personality and pronounced affect blunting, thought disorder, or catatonic stupor, without symptoms of cloudiness or affective features. The schizophreniform, or atypical, schizophrenia, by contrast, is marked by a precipitating factor, an acute onset, a clouded sensorium, and a depressive or neurotic background. Genetic studies by Weiner and Strömgren (1958) showed no greater frequency of schizophrenia in the sibs of the schizophreniform patients than in the general population, indicating a different genetic diathesis. Similar findings have been reported by Mitsuda and co-workers (1967), with clinical and genetic differences reported between the nuclear (typical) and peripheral (atypical) forms.
Attention has also been paid to the concept of schizoid personality. Kallmann (1938) felt such borderline cases might be genetic carriers with inhibited manifestations, or phenocopies with no genetic relationship. Heston (1969) has maintained that if schizoid disorders are grouped with the schizophrenic, a single, autosomal, dominant gene may account for the genetic contribution to the basic inherited trait, advancing as further evidence the fact that both disorders, schizoidia and schizophrenia, occur with equal probability in MZ twins of schizophrenics.
A recent diagnostic concept is that of the schizophrenic spectrum, a group of disorders exhibited, e.g., by the biological children of schizophrenics reared in adoptive homes (Rosenthal and co-workers, 1968). The schizophrenic spectrum encompasses various disorders, including schizophrenia itself and borderline states, schizoid disorders, and inadequate personality.
One use of family studies to distinguish between primary and secondary etiology of schizophrenia among the deaf population of New York State; Schizophrenia expectancy rates in this group were found by Rainer and Kallmann (1959) to be something over 2% higher than some, but equal to other, estimates for the general population (Böök, 1960; Deming, 1968). Among the sibs of deaf schizophrenic patients, the risk figure for schizophrenia for all the sibs was found by Altshuler and Sarlin (1962), to be 11.6%; for hearing sibs alone, 11,2%; and for deaf sibs alone, 15.8%. These rates are not significantly different from each other, nor from the 14.3% rate found in Kallmann's (1946) study of sibs of schizophrenic index cases without a hearing loss. These data imply that schizophrenia among the totally deaf is not secondary to the deafness. Finally in a classic study of schizophrenia-like psychoses of epilepsy the patients showed a generally downhill course, but the risk of schizophrenia in first-degree relatives was no greater than in the general population (Slater and co-workers, 1963).
Theses genetic investigations (family, twin and adoption) over many decades can provide the research investigator with a sophistication in diagnostic evaluation; this sophistication is essential for the clinician and indispensable for the genetic counselor. To have read about or seen twin pairs with greatly differing grades of symptoms, to have studies, e.g., the story of the Genain quadruplets (Rosenthal,

1963), can give the counselor a feeling for the "norm of reaction" of the schizophrenic genotype and temper his prognoses. Roberts (1963) believes that "genetic advice on mental disease must be left to psychiatrists. Some of those interviewed, and the histories they give, need psychiatric appraisal. What is even more important is the difficulty to anyone not a psychiatrist of interpreting and assessing psychiatric reports". A second contribution of psychiatry to genetic counseling concerns ways of presenting material and discussing it with persons who need help (Rainer, 1967).

Armed with clinical experience and the added knowledge derived from studying families, twins, adopted children, and high-risk children from early childhood on, the psychiatrist-counselor can provide responsible and sound advice to accompany improvements in treatment in homes where schizophrenia is present. Marriage choice, family planning, child rearing, adoption, and foster care are all questions that fall under the wider sphere of genetic counseling (Rainer, 1969).

Empirically, risks run from about 40% in the children of two schizophrenic parents to about 15% in children of one schizophrenic parent; the theoretical risks of 100% in the former case under a recessive theory or 50% in the latter under a dominant have not been observed. Since most persons do not consider risks below 10% to be serious, the clearest indication for a warning of caution is in the case of dual matings; with one parent affected, the empirical risk for the offspring is low, though not negligible. It is necessary in such cases to help the family consider as equally important in their decision, first, the effect of having a child on the course of illness in the disabled parent, and, second, the effect of a possibly disrupted home on the development of the child regardless of genetic considerations. In all cases, the psychiatrically trained genetic counselor will have the opportunity to utilize all of his diagnostic abilities, psychological understanding, clinical experience, and biological sophistication in dealing with the many family problems presented by schizophrenia. This multidisciplinary approach can best be utilised in longitudinal studies of high risk children.

REFERENCES

Abrams, R., M. Taylor, and P. Gaztanaga (1974). Arch. Gen. Psychiat., 31, 640-642.
Altshuler, K.Z., and B. Sarlin (1962). In F.J.Kallmann (Ed.), Expanding Goals of Genetics in Psychiatry, Grune and Stratton, New York. pp. 52-62.
Angst, J. (1966). Monogr. Gesamtgeb. Psychiatr., 112, Berlin.
Asano, N. (1967). In H. Mitsuda (Ed.), Clinical Genetics in Psychiatry, Bunkosha Co Ltd, Kyoto. pp. 262-275.
Belmaker, R.H., and R.J. Wyatt (1974). (Personal communication).
Böök, J.A. (1953). Acta Genet., 4, 1-100.
Böök, J.A. (1960). Milbank Mem. Fund. Q., 38, 193-212.
Brown, R.J., R.C. Elston, W.S. Pollitzer, A. Prange, and I. Wilson (1973). Biol. Psychiat., 6, 307-309.
Clayton, P.J., L. Rodin, and G. Winokur (1968). Compr. Psychiat., 9, 31-49.
Cohen, S.M., M.G. Allen, W. Pollin, and H. Hrubec (1972). Arch. Gen. Psychiat., 26, 539-546.
Cooper, J.E., R.E. Kendall, B.J. Gurland, L. Sharp, J.R.M. Copeland, and R. Simon (1972). Psychiatric Diagnosis in New York and London, Oxford Univ. Press, London.
Crowe, R.R., and P.E. Smouse (1974). (Personal communication).
Da Fonseca, A.F. (1959). Analise heredo-clinica das perturbacoes affectivas, Dissertation, University of Porto.
Deming, W.E. (1968). Behav. Sci., 13, 467-476.
Elsasser, G. (1952). Die Nachkommen geistaskranker Elternpaare, Thieme, Stuttgart.
Fialkow, P.J., E.R. Giblett, and A.G. Motulsky (1967). Am. J. Hum. Genet., 19, 63-67.
Garmezy, N. (1965). In M.M. Katz, J.O. Cole, and W.E. Barton (Eds.), Classification in Psychiatry and Psychopathology, US Govt. Printing Office, Washington

D.C. pp. 419-466.
Goetzl, V., R. Green, P. Whybrow, and R. Jackson (1974). Arch. Gen. Psychiat., 31, 665-672.
Gottesman, I.I., and J. Schields (1972). Schizophrenia and Genetics: A Twin Study Vantage Point, Academic Press, New York.
Harvald, B., and M. Hauge (1965). In J.V. Neel, M.W. Shaw, and W.J. Schull (Eds.). Genetics and the Epidemiology of Chronic Diseases, US Dept of Health, Education and Welfare, Washington D.C. pp. 61-76.
Helgasson, T. (1964). Acta Psychiat. Scand, Suppl. 173, 1-258.
Heston, L.L. (1969). Science, 167, 249-256.
Kallmann, F.J. (1938). The Genetics of Schizophrenia, Augustin, New York.
Kallmann, F.J. (1946). Am. J. Psychiat., 103,309-322.
Kallmann, F.J. (1954). In P. Hoch, and J. Zubin (Eds.), Depression, Grune and Stratton, New York. pp. 1-24.
Kidd, K.K., and L.L. Cavalli-Sforza (1973). Social Biology, 20, 254-265.
Kringlen, E. (1967). Heredity and Environment in the Functional Psychoses. An Epidemiological-Clinical Twin Study, Universitstoforlaget, Oslo.
Kringlen, E. (1968). In D. Rosenthal, and S. Kety (Eds.), The Transmission of Schizophrenia, Pergamon Press, Oxford. pp. 49-64.
Langfeldt, G. (1939). The Schizophreniform States, Oxford Univ. Press, London.
Leonhard, K. (1959). Aufteilung der endogenen Psychosen, Akademie-Verlag, Berlin.
Lewis, A. (1967). Inquiries on Psychiatry, Science House, New York.
Mendlewicz, J., J.L. Fleiss, and R.R. Fieve (1972a). JAMA, 222, 1627.
Mendlewicz, J., R.R. Fieve, J.D. Rainer, and J.L. Fleiss (1972b). Br. J. Psychiat., 120, 523-530.
Mendlewicz, J., R.R. Fieve, J.D. Rainer, and M. Cataldo (1973). Br. J. Psychiat., 122, 31-34.
Mendlewicz, J., and J.L. Fleiss (1974). Biol. Psychiat., 9, 261-294.
Mendlewicz, J., and J.D. Rainer (1974). Am. J. Hum. Genet., 26, 692-701.
Mendlewicz, J., T. Massart Gniot, J. Wilmotte, and J.L. Fleiss (1974). Dis. Nerv. Syst., 35, 39-41.
Mendlewicz, J., and J.D. Rainer (1977). Nature, 268, 327-329.
Mendlewicz, J., J.L. Fleiss, and R.R. Fieve (In Press). In R.R. Fieve, D.Rosenthal and H. Brill (Eds.), Genetics and Psychopathology, John Hopkins Press, Baltimore MD.
Ministry of Health (1969). Patient Statistics from the Mental Health Enquiry for the Years 1964, 1965 and 1966, H.M. Stationery Office, Statistical Report Series n° 4, London.
Mitsuda, H. (1967). Clinical Genetics in Psychiatry, Igaku-Shoin, Tokyo.
Parker, J.B., A. Theillie, and C.D. Spielberger (1961). J. Ment. Sci., 107, 936-942.
Perris, C. (1968). Acta Psychiat. Scand., Suppl. 203, 45-52.
Perris, C. (1972). Br. J. Psychiat., 118, 207-210.
Price, J. (1968). In A.Coppen, and A. Walk (Eds.), Recent Developments in Affective Disorders, Br. J. Psychiat., Spec. Publ. n° 2, London.
Rainer, J.D., and F.J. Kallmann (1959). In B. Pasamanick (Ed.), Epidemiology of Mental Disorder, Am. Assoc. of the Advancement of Science, Washington D.C. pp. 229-247.
Rainer, J.D. (1967). In J. Masserman (Ed.), Current Psychiatric Therapies, Vol. 7, Grune and Stratton, New York. pp. 82-91.
Rainer, J.D. (1969). In F. Redlich (Ed.), Social Psychiatry, Williams and Wilkins, Baltimore MD. pp. 222-229.
Reich, T., P.J. Clayton, and G. Winokur (1969). Am. J. Psychiat., 125, 1358-1359.
Renwick, J.H., and J. Schulze (1964). Am. J. Hum. Genet., 16, 410-418.
Roberts, J.A.F. (1963). An Introduction to Medical Genetics, Oxford Univ. Press, London.
Rosanoff, A.H., L.M. Handy, and I.B.A. Rosanoff-Plesset (1934). Am. J. Psychiat., 91, 752-762.

Rosenthal, D. (1963). The Genain Quadruplets, Basic Books, New York.
Rosenthal, D., P.H. Wender, S.S. Kety, F. Schulsinger, J. Welner, and L.Ostergaard (1968). In D. Rosenthal, and S. Kety (Eds.), Transmission of Schizophrenia, Pergamon Press, Oxford. pp. 377-391.
Rüdin, E. (1923). Z. Ges. Neurol. Psychiatr., 81, 459-496.
Schultz, B. (1940). Z. Ges. Neurol. Psychiatr., 170, 441-514.
Schultz, B., and K. Leonhardt (1940). Z. Ges. Neurol. Psychiatr., 168, 587-613.
Sjögren, J. (1948). Acta Psychiat. Scand., Suppl. 52.
Slater, E. (1953). Psychotic and Neurotic Illness in Twins, Spec. Rep. Ser. Med. Res. Coun. 278, HM Stationery Office, London.
Slater, E., A.W. Beard, and F. Glithero (1963). Br. J. Psychiat., 109, 95-150.
Slater, E., J. Maxwell, and J.S. Price (1972). Br. J. Psychiat., 118, 215-218.
Smith, J.C. (1925). J. Nerv. Ment. Dis., 62, 1-32.
Stenstedt, A. (1952). Acta Neurol. Psychiat. Scand, Suppl. 79.
Strömgren, E. (1938). Beitrage zur psychiatrischen Erblehere, Munksgaard, Copenhagen.
Strömgren, S. (1965). Acta Psychiat. Scand., 41, 483-489.
Taylor, M., and R. Abrams (1974). Arch. Gen. Psychiat., 28, 656-672.
Tomasson, H. (1938). Acta Psychiat. Neurol. Scand., 13, 517-526.
Weiner, J., And E. Strömgren (1958). Acta Psychiat. Neurol. Scand., 33, 377-399.
Winokur, G., and V.L. Tanna (1969). Dis. Nerv. Syst., 30, 89-94.
Winokur, G., P.J. Clayton, and T. Reich (1969). Manic-Depressive Illness, Mosby, St Louis, Missouri.
Zerbin-Rüdin, E. (1967). In P.E. Becker (Ed.), Human-Genetik: ein kurzes Handbuch in fünf Bänden, Vol. 2, Thieme, Stuttgard. pp. 446-557.
Zerbin-Rüdin, E. (1969). In H. Hippius, and H. Selbach (Eds.), Das depressive Syndrom, Urban and Schwarzenberg, München. pp. 35-56.

Affective Disorders and ABO Blood Types: a Critical Review

P. Rinieris and C. Stefanis

Department of Psychiatry, University of Athens, Eginition Hospital, Athens, Greece

ABSTRACT

The studies on the association between affective disorders (bipolar affective disorder, unipolar affective disorder and involutional melancholia) and ABO blood types are reviewed and discussed.

KEYWORDS

Bipolar affective disorder; unipolar affective disorder; involutional melancholia; ABO blood types.

INTRODUCTION

A number of studies on the association between affective disorders and ABO blood types have yielded conflicting results. The discrepancy might be attributed to several factors, such as differences between individual investigators and departments with respect to the diagnostic criteria, and variations in blood group distribution among populations living in different geographic areas. An additional and probably important factor might be the small number of the investigated patients in the majority of these studies, a disadvantage that would concequently allow for the random formation of the results.
With regard to bipolar affective disorder, positive associations between this disorder and blood type AB (Diebold,1976), blood type A (Flemenbaum and Larson, 1976) or blood type O (Parker and co-workers, 1961; Masters, 1967; Mendlewicz and co-workers, 1974; Shapiro and co-workers, 1977; Rinieris and co-workers, 1979; Singh and co-workers, 1979) have been reported. Other studies failed to reveal any relation between this disorder and ABO blood types (Thomas and Hewitt, 1939; Bourgeois and Tréjaut, 1967; Gaekwad and co-workers, 1972; James and co-workers, 1977). Taking into account the fact that bipolar affective disorder poses less serious diagnostic problems than other affective disorders (since only an episode of mania or hypomania and an episode of depression are - by definition - required for the diagnosis of bipolar affective disorder), the studies on the association between bipolar affective disorder and ABO blood types must not have differences with respect to the diagnostic criteria. The latter possibly accounts for the agreement on the results obtained in half (six) of these studies. Thus, the over-representation of blood group O in patients with bipolar affective disorder, which has been independently found by six groups of investigators in different geographic areas, might be considered as the most replicable finding in this area of research.

With regard to unipolar affective disorder, positive associations between this disorder and blood type A (Shapiro and co-workers, 1977) or blood type O (Rinieris and co-workers, 1979) have been reported, whereas other studies failed to reveal any relation between this disorder and ABO blood types (James and co-workers, 1979; Singh and co-workers, 1979). Not surprisingly there were differences between the above groups of investigators with respect to the criteria used for the diagnosis of unipolar affective disorder. Thus, to be considered as suffering from unipolar affective disorder, it was required that the past history was negative for mania or hypomania and that the patients had had one or more episodes of depression (James and co-workers, 1979), at least two definite episodes of depression (Singh and co-workers, 1979), at least three definite (or two definite and one possible) episodes of depression (Shapiro and co-workers, 1977), and at least three definite episodes of depression (Rinieris and co-workers, 1979). Another probable source of discrepancy between the results of these studies, might have been the small number of the investigated patients in the majority of these studies, which might consequently have led to random formation of the results. Thus, only 23 unipolar depressed patients were investigated by Shapiro and co-workers (1977), 31 by James and co-workers (1979), 43 by Rinieris and co-workers (1979) and 96 patients by Singh and co-workers (1979). In conclusion, a study on the association between unipolar affective disorder and ABO blood types, in which, however, the diagnosis would lay on more stringent criteria (e.g. at least three definite episodes of depression and lack of episodes of mania or hypomania) and in which a significant number of patients would be investigated, would be more than welcome.

With regard to involutional melancholia, positive associations between this disorder and blood type O (Irvine and Miyashita, 1965) or blood type A (Rinieris and co-workers, 1979) have been found, whereas another study failed to reveal any relation between this disorder and ABO blood types (Masters, 1967). This discrepancy might be attributed to the relatively small numbers of the investigated patients in the three studies (i.e., 34 patients were investigated by Irvine and Miyashita (1965), 56 patients by Masters (1967) and 60 patients by Rinieris and co-workers (1979)) and to the fact that Masters' (1967) sample consisted not only of patients with involutional melancholia, but of patients with senile depression, too. It would be, perhaps, of some value to add that Rinieris and co-workers (1979) reported that with respect to ABO blood type distribution pattern, the group of patients with involutional malancholia differed significantly not only from the groups of patients with bipolar or unipolar affective disorder, but differed also from a subgroup of 34 patients with bipolar or unipolar affective disorder with illness' onset after age 40. These findings might be considered as suggesting that the genetic loading in patients with involutional melancholia is different from that in patients with bipolar or unipolar affective disorder. The same conclusion might be drawn from family investigations of patients with involutional melancholia, which showed that - contrary to what holds for bipolar and unipolar depressed patients - probands with involutional melancholia are less likely to have a family history of affective disorder in their first degree relatives, as compared to controls who were in the same age range (Majer, 1941; Stenstedt, 1959).

REFERENCES

Bourgeois, M., and N. Tréjaut (1967). Ann. Méd. Psychol., 125, 447-450.
Diebold, K. (1976). Arch. Psychiat. Nervenkr., 222, 257-265.
Flemenbaum, A., and J.W. Larson (1976). Dis. Nerv. Syst., 37, 581-583.
Gaekwad, R.S., A.K. Niyogi, and R. Jagtiani (1972). Indian J. Med. Sci., 26, 493-495.
Irvine, D.G., and H. Miyashita (1965). Canad. Med. Ass. J., 92, 551-554.
James, N.McI., B.J. Carroll, R.F. Haines, and P.E. Smouse (1979). In J. Mendlewicz and B. Shopsin (Eds.) Genetic Aspects of Affective Illness. Spectrum Publications Inc., New York. pp. 35-44.

Majer, O. (1941). Zeit. Neurol. Psychiat., 172, 737-742.
Masters, A.B. (1967). Br. J. Psychiat., 113, 1309-1315.
Mendlewicz, J., T. Massart-Guiot, J. Wilmotte, and J.L.Fleiss (1974). Dis. Nerv. Syst., 35, 39-41.
Parker, J.B., A. Theilie, and C.D. Spielberger (1961). J. Ment. Sci., 107, 936-942.
Rinieris, P.M., C.N. Stefanis, E.P. Lykouras, and E.K. Varsou (1979). Acta Psychiat. Scand., 60, 272-278.
Shapiro, R.W, O.J. Rafaelsen, L.P. Ryder, A. Svejgaard, and H. Sorensen (1977). Am. J. Psychiat., 134, 197-200.
Singh, G., M.L. Agrawal, J.S. Sachdeva, and A.K. Gupta (1979). Indian J. Psychiat., 21, 80-83
Stenstedt, A. (1959). Acta Psychiat. Neurol. Scand. (Suppl. 127), 34, 1-71.
Thomas, J.C., and E.J.C. Hewitt (1939). J. Ment. Sci., 85, 667-688.

Comparative Investigation of Two Pairs of Monozygotic Twins, One With and the Other Without Endogenous Depression

B. Alevizos, A. Kokkevi, M. Markianos and C. Stefanis

Department of Psychiatry, University of Athens, Eginition Hospital, Athens, Greece

ABSTRACT

Two pairs of monozygotic twins, genetically predisposed to depression, one pair being free of any clinical symptomatology of mental disorder and the other concordant for endogenous depression, have been subjected to an intensive clinical, psychological and neurochemical investigation. The results obtained from this investigation have shown that there are interpair and intrapair similarities and differences which however do not follow a consistent pattern that could pathogenetically be linked to the clinical manifestation of depressive disorder in patient twins.

KEYWORDS

Monozygotic twins; depression.

INTRODUCTION

Detailed family investigations as well as extensive twin and adoption studies have yielded additional evidence to corroborate the hypothesis of a genetic contribution to the affective disorders of the manic-depressive type (for review see Mendlewicz in this volume). It is though still unclear to which psychological, behavioral or biological features of the individual this genetic vulnerability is associated with, as it is equally unclear which of the environmental factors may be most instrumental in activating the predisposed individual to become affectively ill. One research strategy that might yield some useful information in this area would be the in depth and global investigation of a population of monozygotic (MZ) twin pairs comprising all possible variations: Healthy pairs free from any genetic loading for affective disorders. Healthy pairs genetically predisposed for affective disorders. One pair-member affectively ill and the other not (discordant for affective disorder) with or without genetic predisposition. Both pair-members affectively ill (concordant for affective disorder) with or without genetic predisposition. Sorting our intrapair and interpair similarities and differences we might be able to acquire a deeper insight into the intricate play of genes and environmental forces which shapes behavior and determines the various aspects of clinical depression. In this paper we will present the preliminary findings of such an investigation of two pairs of MZ twins both being genetically predisposed to depression but only the twins of one of the two pairs having already manifested depressive episodes.

MATERIAL AND METHODS

Case reports

a) Healthy twins: They are female 23 year old medical students, the only children of a middle class family. They look identical in appearance, they have the same tooth conformation, hair colour and nailbed structure. To others their behaviour is indistinguishable, but according to their self-description they are 80% alike and 20% different in character.

Twin A is described as more conscientious and obsessive, while twin V is described as more extrovert and sociable. The parents are referred to as ordinary people, happily adjusted to their role assignment in the family without any overt interpersonal conflict. Their father now age 55, had two major depressive episodes, the first at the age of 28 and the second at the age of 42.

b) Twins concordant for depression: They are female 20 years old, Law school students, the only children of a middle class family. They are identical in appearence, voice, tooth conformation and nailbed structure. Their behaviour appears strikingly similar and according to them even relatives find it difficult to distinguish one from the other. The father describes himself as basically depressive who rarely feels happy and optimistic. Obsessive, very particular about details and extremely careful not to make anybody angry at him, he held a submissive role in the family. He had 3-4 major depressive episodes which were successfully treated by antidepressant drugs. The mother is overanxious with a tendency to dramatize ordinary situations, in many respects hysterical and unequivoqually the leading person in the family. She often resorts to minor tranquillizers to cope with excessive anxiety and facilitate sleep. Regarding the personality of the twins descriptions by the parents and the twins themselves indicate that until the age of seven R was considered to be the extrovert, the initiator of social contacts and in general the dominant figure of the twins. Following that age a gradual change has taken place in the reverse direction. R became more introverted, more conscientious and reserved, while K replaced R in her previous leading role. This was crystalized at the age of ten and ever since remains unaltered. Their scholastic aptitude was rated equal for both by parents and themselves. They both acknowledge the fact that although they were talked into entering the Law School by their parents, they are artistically inclined and they would prefer to become professional artists. They are currently taking courses in painting while they are attending Law School. They are both quite feminine and attractive girls and they were flirting with boys since their teens. They had sexual relations at the age of 19, but according to their account they feel awkward with boys, passive and submissive. Dependency needs and conformity to social environment were particularly pronounced in R's social behaviour.

In Sept. 1978 K, while she was 18, without any apparent reason started not feeling well and soon she developped a typical depression with psychomotor retardation, a-

Comparative Investigation of Two Pairs of Monozygotic Twins

version to work, pessimism, insomnia, helplessness, feelings of inadequacy and guilt and persistent suicidal thoughts. Five months later without special treatment she started feeling better and by the end of the 6th month the depressive episode had subsided completely and K resumed her regular activities. While K was on her 2nd month of depression, R developped a similar depression, the only difference being a more rapid development and a longer duration (8 months). They were both free of any symptoms only for a few months. In late August 1979, K had a relapse and two months later R followed. It was at that time that they were advised to consult our Outpatient Clinic and their investigation started.

Investigative procedure

Following a stardardized psychiatric interview twin pairs were rated for severity of their depression by using Hamilton's, Zung's, V. Zerssen's and Beck's scales. Zung's Anxiety Scale and Holme's and Rahe's Recent Life Events Questionnaire were also used. Psychological assessment included the MMPI, the Fould's Hostility and Direction of Hostility Questionnaire (H.D.H.Q.), Navran's Dependency Scale (Dy), the Eysenck's Personality Inventory (E.P.I.).Rorschach's test and the Wechsler Intelligence Scale (W.A.I.S.). All psychological tests related to personality investigation in patient twins were performed at a time that no symptomatology was clinically evident. In addition to routine laboratory examinations the following biochemical parameters were investigated: Plasma dopamine-b-hydroxylase (DBH), platelet and plasma monoaminoxidase (MAO), platelet and plasma γ-glutamyl transpeptidase (γ-GT) and plasma cyclic AMP concentrations. All blood samples were taken at a fixed hour in the morning (8.30 a.m.).

In patient twins the plasma level of a single dose of chlomipramine (initially of 25mg and after 3 days of 100 mg) was determined before the onset of regular treatment.

Course of the illness and response to treatment were evaluated by regular, on a weekly basis, clinical assessment and depression and anxiety rating scales were completed.

RESULTS

The findings of the present investigation appear in tables, in which the patient twins are represented by A1 (K) and A2 (R), while the healthy-twins are represented by B1 (A) and B2 (V).

The results obtained from the Eysenck's and the Fould's Hostility and Direction of Hostility Questionnaires are shown in table 1. There are some strong intrapair similarities (in P and E in the Eysenck in the patient pair, in AH, CO, G in the Fould's questionnaire in the healthy pair) but some pronounced differences as well. The most striking intrapair difference was in the direction of hostility.

TABLE 1 Results of the E.P.I. and H.D.H.Q. in Two Pairs of Monozygotic Twins.

A) Eysenck's Personality Questionnaire

	P	N	E	L
A1	3	8	15	11
A2	3	11	15	6
B1	3	16	9	13
B2	7	12	11	15

B) Foul's Hostility and Direction of Hostility Questionnaire

	AH	CO	DH	SC	G	Direction*
A1	5	8	3	7	5	+8
A2	10	9	10	2	1	-14
B1	3	2	0	0	1	-3
B2	3	2	2	3	2	+3

* + introverted
  - extraverted

The MMPI profile of the twin-patients is not identical but not strikingly different either. Dependency scores are quite high for both, but is higher by ten points in the twin that also shows a more pronounced psychopathology. The MMPI profile of the healthy twin was not identical, but the intrapair differences were minimal (table 2).

TABLE 2 MMPI Findings

	Profile	Dy scale score
A1 : 872140' 639*	38
A2 : 81' 92307	29
B1 : '248	32
B2 : Normal range	23

*1. Hypochondriasis; 2. Depression; 3. Hysteria; 4. Psychopathic deviation; 6. Paranoia; 7. Psychasthenia; 8. Schizophrenia; 9. Mania, 0. Social Introversion; 'upper normal limit.

The I.Q. scores for the two pairs of twins are shown in table 3. Intrapair differences exist, but they are minor.

TABLE 3 I.Q. Scores (W.A.I.S.)

	Full Scale	Verbal	Perform.
A1	101	111	99
A2	96	102	90
B1	112	125	94
B2	106	119	89

Comparative Investigation of Two Pairs of Monozygotic Twins   21

In the Rorschach's test the main common characteristic for the healthy twins were signs of neurotic personality and intense sexual preoccupation. Responses given by B2 provide additional indication of a highly inhibited person with intense internal conflicts. Somatic preoccupation, depressive and obsessive-compulsive trends were also found to be much more pronounced in B2 than in B1. In patient twins insecurity has been found to be the main common trait. The following additional differential characteristics may also be noted. A1: Extroverted, impulsive, imaginative, creative and narcissistic, prone to anxiety and frustration due to unrealized needs with a tendency towards passive resignation. A2: Dependent, passive, highly self-controlled, phobic, with a tendency towards depression and repression of internal conflicts.

The results from the biochemical investigation are shown in table 4.

TABLE 4 Enzyme Activity of DBH, γ-GT and MAO and cAMP Concentration in MZ Twins.

	DBH nmol/ml	Plasma cAMP pmol/ml	Plasma γ-GT mU/ml	Plat.γ-GT mU/mg	Plat. MAO dpm/mg/30min
A1	29.2	10.25	4.48		
A2	28.6	16.50	3.61		
B1	13.6	18.70	4.16	2.92	5178
B2	17.7	17.60	3.23	2.24	9250

Plasma DBH levels were almost identical in the patient twin pair. They were much lower and not far apart from each other in the healthy twin pair: Plasma cAMP concentrations were almost identical in the healthy twin pair and they differed between the patient twins. The plasma γ-Gt was found markedly low in both pairs with only small intrapair differences. Results from MAO activity determination are presently available only from the healthy twin pair. As can be seen in table 4 MAO's activity values are not similar in the healthy twins.

The results from scoring symptom intensity by various anxiety and depression measuring tools, are shown in table 5.

TABLE 5 Scores in Depression, Anxiety and Life Events Scales

	Zung Anxiety	Zung Depression	Hamilton Depression	V. Zerssen Depression	Holme's and Rahe's Life Events
A1	57	58	22	55	253
A2	55	56	23	44	284
B1	23	25	7		57
B2	33	28	3		114

The scoring for the patient twin pair is very close for both anxiety and depression. The healthy twin pair had low scores for anxiety and even lower for depression. In the Life Events Questionnaire, patient-twins had high and close to each other scores, whereas healthy-twins had low and not close to each other scores.

The clinical course of depression in the twin patients during the first three weeks of chlomipramine treatment is shown in table 6.

TABLE 6 Response to Treatment with Chlomipramine

Scale		Pre-treat.	1st week	2nd week	3rd week
Hamilton	A1	22	11	5	2
	A2	23	16	12	17
Beck	A1	20	10	0	0
	A2	15	7	6	3
Zung Anxiety	A1	57	39	35	28
	A2	55	44	40	20
Zung Depression	A1	58	46	36	31
	A2	56	50	47	41
V. Zerssen	A1	55	2	1	1
	A2	44	7	7	8

Even under treatment the course of the illness was in several ways similar to the previous depressive episode in which no drugs were given. The twin sister A1 who preceded A2 in depressive symptoms by two months, responded better and 6 weeks following treatment she was feeling normal and a substantial decrease in dosage was decided. A2 on the other hand responded very slowly to treatment and by the end of the 6th week of treatment she was still feeling depressed and it was decided that she should increase rather than decrease the antidepressants.

In single dose administration of chlomipramine, particularly at the 100 mg dose, the same plasma level was reached in both sisters indicating a similar in both metabolism of the antidepressant drug (table 7)

TABLE 7. Dose and Plasma Level (ng/ml) of Chlomipramine

Dose (mg)		50	100
Plasma level	A1	38.1	171.4
	A2	27.6	171.4

DISCUSSION

Several attempts based on the twin method were made in the past to determine the heritability of various personality traits. These attempts were only partly successful since studies in which the same methodology was used, yielded conflicting and largely inconclusive results. It is, however, agreed by most authors that certain personality features are more heritable than others. Using the California Psychological Inventory (CPI) in MZ and DZ twins a great number of investigators have found evidence of a differential heritability of personality traits. Carey and co-workers (1978) concluded that the extraversion-introversion factors are the most heritable. Others (Horn and co-workers, 1976) considered factors such as Conversational Poise, Compulsiveness and Social Ease are mostly determined by genes, while Confidence in Leadership, Impulse Control, Philosophical Attitudes, Intellectual Interests, and Exhibitionism are mostly determined by environment. Neuroticism in the Eysenck's Personality Inventory has also been found to be part of the genetic architecture associated with an evolutionary history of stabilizing selection (Eaves and Eysenck, 1976). The same authors attributed the within subjects variation in neuroticism score over a period between tests to environmental factors specific to individuals. It has also been shown that greater resemblance in appearance in identical twins does not make them more similar in personality (Plomin and co-workers, 1976).

To enrich the information regarding the differential share of heredity and environment to personality traits and psychopathology, a number of studies have been carried out in recent years to investigate possible relationships of biochemical parameters and personality characteristics in normal controls and mental patients.

In accordance with the prevailing monoamine hypothesis of the functional psychoses most investigators have focused their attention on enzymes which are closely related to catecholamine metabolism and are largely genetically determined. There is evidence (Nies and co-workers, 1973) that MAO activity is greatly influenced by genetic factors, and low MAO activity has been associated with increased vulnerability to depression (Murphy and Weiss, 1972), with mental disorders in general (Buchsbaum and co-workers, 1976) and even with certain personality traits in normals (Murphy and co-workers, 1977). The evidence that DBH activity is genetically determined is even more convincing (Weinshilboum and co-workers, 1975). This enzyme's activity levels have found to be weakly correlated only with bipolar illness and not with any other mental disorder (Shopsin and co-workers, 1972; Kopin and co-workers, 1976; Levitt and co-workers, 1976; Lerner and co-workers, 1978; Strandman and co-workers, 1978). Winter and co-workers (1978) studied recently the relationships of DBH, MAO and COMT with MMPI scores in a number of MZ and DZ twins and some significant correlations were found between DBH activity and MMPI scores. cAMP plasma concentrations were found low in depression (Lykouras and co-workers, 1978; Stefanis and co-workers, 1979) and it has been claimed that brain cAMP concentrations are genetically determined and associated with the tendency for aggressive attacks (Orenberg and co-workers, 1975). The γ-GT activity has not been extremely studied in relation to mental disorders and particularly to affective illness. It was found to be lower in the leucocytes of schizophrenics compared to controls (Alevizos and Stefanis, 1980).

In the light of the preceding background information, an interpair comparative analysis of our findings does not seem to provide us with any information which would allow us even to speculate on the reasons why depression was elicited in both members of one twin-pair and not in the members of the other pair, although both pairs did not substantially differ in their genetic loading, in their upbringing and in their social and cultural environment. There are though some differences between the pairs which might be of some significance. One difference lies in the MMPI profile. Both patient twins, at a time that no psychopathology was clinically evident, scored in the MMPI psychopathology scales substantially higher than the healthy twins. This might suggest that even in the absence of clinical symptoms, the MMPI profile may be of value in ascertaining vulnerability to depression or other mental disorder. Another interpair difference worth mentioning is the difference in the score of recent life events. Both patient twins had a substantially higher score and this may indicate that in individuals who derive from their genes a cognitive and affective vulnerability, stressful life events may play an important role in precipitating depressive illness. Our findings from the biochemical investigation could hardly be associated with the occurence of depression. The plasma DBH activity was found to be higher in patient than healthy twins. Serum γ-GT activity was rather low but almost identical in both pairs. The same applies to to cAMP plasma concentrations. It is also evident from our findings that there is no clear intrapair and interpair correlation between the biochemical parameters that have been studied. This has already been pointed out by Winter and co-workers, (1978). Considering the fact that intrapair differences in monozygotic twins signify environmental interference, our findings taken together can only allow us to simply state that genetic as well as environmental factors seem to be relevant in the occurence of affective illness. This conclusion is consistent with everyday's clinical experience as well as with systematic studies in which the twin strategy was used (Allen and co-workers, 1974).

At our present state of knowledge and investigative methodology is very unlikely that we may be in a position to precisely evaluate the differential contribution of the many factors to a psychopathological condition such as depression, which, despite certain common characteristics that justify a group-labeling, may not be alike between the affected individuals. Clinical diagnosis may be too broad a concept to be precisely correlated with elementary psychological and biological variables. The need for studying a large set of variables in relation with a mental illness, a phenomenon that is manifested at the highest level of functional integration is to be considered in future research. Such an investigation may greatly be facilitated if it is combined with prospective twin and family studies. From such a global approach based on comparative study of large groups of patients and normals with different degrees of genetic and environmental homogeneity, a consistent pattern of comprehensive relationships rather than straight-line correlations may emerge.

REFERENCES

Alevizos, B.H., and C.N. Stefanis (1980). Neuropsychobiology, 6, 333-340.
Allen, M., S. Cohen, W. Pollin, and S. Greenspan (1974). Am. J. Psychiat., 131, 1234-1239.
Buchsbaum, M.S., D.L. Coursey, and D.L. Murphy (1976). Science, 194, 339-341.
Carey, G., H.H. Goldsmith, A. Tellegen, and I.I. Gottesman (1978). Beh. Genet., 8, 299-313.
Eaves, L., and H. Eysenck (1976). Beh. Genet., 6, 145-160.
Horn, J.M., R. Plomin, and R.Rosenman (1976). Beh. Genet., 6, 17-30.
Kopin, I.J., S. Kaufman, H. Viveros, D. Jacobowitz, C. Lake, M. Ziegler, W.M. Lovenberg, and F.K. Goodwin (1976). Ann. Intern. Med., 85, 211-223.
Lerner, P., F.K. Goodwin, D.P. van Kammen, R.M. Post, L.F. Major, J.C. Ballenger, and W. Lovenberg (1978). Biol. Psychiat., 13, 685-694.
Levitt, M., D.L. Dunner, J. Mendlewicz, D.B. Frewin, W. Lawlor, J.L. Fleiss, F. Stallone, and R.R. Fieve (1976). Psychopharmacologia (Berl.), 46, 205-210.
Lykouras, E., E. Varsou, E. Garelis, C.N. Stefanis, and D. Malliaras (1978). Acta Psychiat. Scand., 57, 447-453.
Murphy, D.L., and R. Weiss (1972). Am. J. Psychiat., 128, 1351-1357.
Murphy, D.L., R.H. Belmaker, M. Buchsbaum, N.F. Martin, R.Cianarello, and R.J. Wyatt (1977). Psychol. Med., 7, 149-157.
Nies, A., D. Robinson, K. Lamborn, and R.P. Lampert (1973). Arch. Gen. Psychiat., 28, 834-838.
Orenberg, E.K., J. Renson, and G.R. Elliot (1975). Psychopharm. Commun., 1, 99-107.
Plomin, R., L. Willerman, and J.C. Loehlin (1976). Beh. Genet., 6, 43-52.
Shopsin, B., L.S. Freedman, M. Goldstein, and S. Gershon (1972). Psychopharmacologia (Berl.), 27, 11-16.
Stefanis, C.N., E. Lykouras, E. Garelis, and E. Varsou (1979). Biol. Psychiat., 15, 149-154.
Strandman, E., L. Wetterberg, C. Perris, and S.B. Ross (1978). Neuropsychobiology, 4, 248-255.
Weinshilboum, R.M., H.G. Schrott, F. A. Raymond, W.H. Weidman, and L.R. Elveback (1975). Am. J. Hum. Genet., 27, 573-585.
Winter, H., M. Herschel, P. Propping, W. Friedl, and F. Vogel (1978). Psychopharmacology, 57, 63-69.

2. Clinical Aspects of Depression

Psychopathology of Depression

K. Achté

Department of Psychological Medicine, University of Helsinki, Helsinki, Finland

ABSTRACT

In this paper the difficulties in classifying the various types of depression as well as the problems related to differential diagnosis of depression are presented. The psychodynamic mechanisms underlying depressive psychopathology are extensively reviewed and their relevance to current treatment approaches are discussed.

KEYWORDS

Depression; psychodymanic; classification of depression; psychopathology.

INTRODUCTION

In the literature contradictory opinions have been presented as to whether the depressive form of manic-depressive psychosis is indentical with reactive depressive psychosis. Angst and Weiss (1968) have differentiated between unipolar and bipolar disorder manifestations according to the fact whether only depressive or both depressive and manic episodes occur in the patient. Perris (1966) and Angst (1966) present the view that bipolar manic-depressive psychosis is genetically different from unipolar depressive psychosis. Nevertheless, not all researchers hold this stand. For example, Kendell (1968) could not discern any clear-cut difference between manic-depressive psychosis and other depressive psychoses. According to him, the same patient could fall ill with psychoses of different types in the course of her life. Yet it seems plausible that clear-cut and typical manic-depressive psychoses appear in one end of the axis and reactive psychoses in the other. The various disease pictures met with in practical work fall in this continuum in the intervening space between these two end points. The distinction between neurotic and psychotic depression is quite indefinite, and there are numerous transitional forms between the two. Sense of reality is distorted in psychoses. Transcultural aspects of depressions merit special attention.

Forms of depression

Depression appears in many forms. Deep and severe inhibited depression of psychotic level is frequently called endogenous depression. Inhibited depressive psychosis, referring to the typical endogenous depression, implies the following symptoms as a triad: decline of mood, psychomotor inhibition, self-accusations and depressive delusions. Another very common form of depressive psychosis is agitated depressive psychosis. In this disease manifestation inhibition is absent, on the contrary, the patient suffers from severe anxiety which may even lead to expressions of motor restlessness. Depressive disease pictures are often encountered in connection with involutional psychoses.

Another classification of depressions distinguishes between inhibited apathetic, inhibited agitated, neurasthenic-hypochondriac and excited agitated depressions.

Grinker and his collaborators distinguished four types of depressive patients(1961).
1. Hopeless patients whose self-esteem is low but who harbor only very mild feelings of guilt. They tend to be isolated, apathetic and speak slowly. Approximately one third of all patients suffering from depression may be regarded as belonging to this group.
2. Patients who are hopeless. Their self-esteem is low and they exhibit guilt feelings, anxiety and features of agitated depression.
3. Hypochondriac patients who often are agitated. They have only seldom feelings of guilt but they are characterized by the feeling that nobody cares for them.
4. Patients who are hopeless and agitated and in whom aggressiveness and provocative tendencies can be discerned.

Grinker and his team construed these various forms of depression in the way that, considering the patient's personality, each form of depression corresponded to the patient's difficulties, attempts of restitution and to the dominating defense mechanisms of the personality against anxiety and psychic pain.
Ottosson divides depressions into three groups (1969):
1. Endogenous depression
2. Psychogenic depression
3. Somatogenic depression
Endogenous depression was previously regarded as belonging to the category of manic-depressive illness.

Psychogenic depression is usually referred to if the disturbance is associated with reactive factors. Differentiating between neurotic depression is indeterminate and vague. Nevertheless, almost all forms of depression involve in a greater or lesser degree psychological factors which have contributed to the development of the disorder. Somatogenic depression includes a number of depressions associated with organic diseases.
Several additional principles of classification have been applied in characterizing depression. Many of them are essentially dichotomies, the use of which may be considered a tendency to dogmatize and systematize depressions and psychiatry in general.
Neurotic depressions are vastly more common than psychotic depressions. Neuroses are not surveyed in this connection. Alcoholism, drug abuse and sociopathic behavior have often been called slow suicide when the underlying motive has been seen to constitute the patient's effort to overcome depression through such behaviors.
The frequency of suicides among male alcoholics is sixty-fold as compared with male population of the same age and two hundred-fold as compared with the mean population. These figures support the view presented above about indirect suicidal behavior.
The concept of anaclitic depression was introduced into psychiatry by Spitz in the forties (1946). This phenomenon is not infrequent in babies as young as six months who have been separated from their parents, above all from the mother, for a couple of months. These children develop a syndrome resembling endogenous depression. Excitement and crying spells are followed by apathy, indifference, insomnia, fast-

ing and over-all retardation of vital functions. The symptoms disappear if the child is allowed to return to his mother.

Symptoms of depression and its psychology

In depression the patient's superego is unduly strict and rigid. Quite often, when viewing superficially, the patient's premorbid personal relationships appear to have been good and the patient himself seems to have been an extrovert. Yet, his emotional bonds with other people are characterized by ambivalence, and his object relationships may be quite superficial. Depression implies an intensive sense of illness and subjective suffering. The depressive patient is often characterized by fatigue, insomnia, loss of initiative and vitality and a melancholic attitude toward life which frequently includes features of hopelessness. Guilt feelings, diminished self-esteem and anxiety are common symptoms of depression. Motor inhibition is often associated with psychotic depression. Hypochondriac symptoms in depression represent the patient's attempts to find support and transfer of instinctual energy from external objects toward oneself.
Depressive patients complain of dejection, tiredness, fatigue, lack of energy and inability to concentrate. They seem to enjoy nothing. Life appears meaningless and gloomy. Decrease of self-esteem, feelings of inferiority, hopelessness and indifference are components of the symptomatology of depression. The patient cannot force his mood to get higher. The more he tries, the worse he is off. Aches of diverse character are often among the symptoms of depression, likewise common are feelings of restlessness and tension, stomach troubles and dizziness. Very often the patients harbor feelings of guilt. Typical features in psychotic depressions include grave irrealistic self-accusations, inhibition, loss of interest in one's environment and insomnia. In addition to difficulty in falling asleep, depressive insomniac symptoms appear specifically as sleeplessness of the very early hours so that the patient wakes up after having slept only some hours, and typically when awaking some time after midnight he is anxious and agitated. Impotence and irregularities in menstruation or amenorrhoea, dryness of the mouth, obstipation, deep concern for the future, lack of expression or an expression of distress, retardation of motor functions, difficulties in concentrating which subjectively may be experienced as loss of memory, most diverse sensations felt in various parts of the body and a deep sense of illness are characteristic symptoms of psychotic depression.
Latent depression may manifest itself solely in inexplicable decrease in vitality and energy, tiredness and fluctuations of mood. Mood may oscillate by diurnal interchange. Mornings are often distressing and laden with anxiety. The patient may be fretful, weary of life and afraid of various things. The depressive patient's energy is inhibited. It is hard to start the daily pursuits. Appetite is clearly reduced or entirely lost. Life is experienced as absolutely worthless. The mouth gets dry. Particularly in the initial stages of severe depressions there occur very frequently somatic symptoms of psychogenic origin, and similar developments occur also when the depression gets protracted. More mildly depressive patients do not necessarily suffer from any particular somatic symptoms. Sometimes depressive patients exhibit conversion symptoms which may impress the clinical picture. Other common somatic manifestations include tremors and headache. The patient may experience various somatic sensations all over the body as equivalents of anxiety and depression. These symptoms may take the form of paresthesias, pains or sensations of several other types. Vision may get blurred, leading the patient to turn to an ophthalmologist. In a grave depression the whole world may transform so as to appear grey. Typical cutaneous symptoms include itching, very dry skin and paresthesias. In differential diagnosis it is well to bear in mind the possibility of hypothyroidism in which cutaneous symptoms are frequent. Occasionally tachycardia and painful or distressing sensations in the chest are associated with depression. In the agitated stage of depression the patient's blood pressure may rise. Polla-

kisuria or a very frequent need of urination is a common symptom in depression. It
must be remembered that antidepressant drugs, too, exert an anticholinergic action
leading to dryness of the mouth and accommodation disturbances.
Quite often depressions typically involve a depersonalization sensation which makes the patient feel that he cannot any longer love his relatives and close friends like he did before. In milder cases the patient may be troubled by a difficulty in concentration and an inability to manage in his duties in the way he used
to. In severe cases general inhibition and an inability to work at all gradually
emerge. The patient speaks slowly. His whole nature and facial expression become
rigid. Speech grows into a gloomy sound. On objective examination intelligence
and memory are found to be undisturbed. There are no disorders of orientation,
sense of time or thinking faculty.
Many depressions begin with loss of appetite and weight reduction. It is a very
frequent phenomenon that the patient does not complain of depressiveness at all,
but instead declares to suffer from tiredness, inability to concentrate, lack of
energy, weakness and loss of interest. Quite often depressions involve sweating
and symptoms of the autonomic nervous system, loss of lacrimation or crying spells.
The sleep of a person with depression contains unusually few REM phases.
In agitated depression the patient is restless and anxious. If sleep is poor, hypermotility may lead to exhaustive conditions. Psychotic depressions may include
paranoid manifestations and querulous features. For example, the patient may think
that other people despise him or that he is bound to be thrown into jail. Hypochondriac symptoms occur frequently in psychotic depressions, and often they are
of grotesque character. For instance, the patient may claim that he has got no
bowels or brain at all, or he may believe that his veins have dried off.
Obsessive and depressive features frequently occur simultaneously. When depression
has subsided the patient can often still suffer from obsessive-compulsive symptoms. Many persons liable to depressions can be afraid of losing their money. In
such cases money apparently is connected with certain anal aspects. Food is frequently of essential significance, and patients often undergo bulimic episodes.
Warmth has often a precious symbolic meaning for depressive patients while coldness in a way symbolizes distance and coolness in personal relationships.

Psychology of depression

In the year 1911 Abraham published a study of patients with depression he had
treated. According to him, the symptoms and personality of severely depressive,
cyclothymic patients are characterized by the absence of satisfactory, lasting object relationships. Their attitude toward their close persons was hampered by
strong emotional conflicts. In addition to love and dependency they exhibited simultaneously hostility toward their close persons. Guilt feelings and the notion
that they are not loved which arose in the psychotic stage were based on their own
hostility. During the psychotic episode their contacts with the outer world were
partly broken. They were unable to love, and they themselves were aware of this
wherefore they blamed themselves in their self-accusations and guilt feelings.
Depression is characterized by a conflict between hostility and strong yearning of
love. As for premorbid personality, depressive patients are persons who are liked.
Due to their low self-esteem they endeavor to please others in order to acquire
warmth in their personal relationships. It is typical to them that they wish to be
good, strong, powerful, loved and appreciated; they do not want to have the opposite qualities (Bibring 1953). They have set their objectives very high, wherefore
they are difficult to reach, and this again exposes the person to depression. The
difference between the ego and the ego ideal - that is what the person wishes she
were - is often very great in a person who is depressive or liable to depression.
Frequently this wide difference is created as a reaction to hard childhood conditions. The depressive person is unable to make this gap narrower by various reactive mechanisms. He experiences feelings of helplessness and hopelessness, anxie-

ty and depression. Use of tranquilizers and abcohol may temporarily alleviate symptoms, since the sedative effect of the drug refuces agressiveness, thereby diminishing guilt feelings and elevating self-esteem for a while. So the patient may feel a bit more satisfied with himself. The patient endeavors to mitigate his feelings of guilt and worthlessness by means of various defence mechanisms of the ego. Psychoanalytic study has promoted researches concerning psychology of depression. Depression involves features of the oral stage of psychosexual development. Grief and depression have many common characteristics. If the person loses a loved object, grief sets in. During the process called the work of mourning the emotional load or libido fixed onto this loved object is gradually detached from its original object being transferred onto new objects. This is hard, indeed, but absolutely necessary in regard to the fact that life must go on. The length of the period of mourning depends on the situation and the strength of the emotional bond. The period of mourning following the death of a close person lasts as an intensive feelingfrom half a year to two years. Grief often involves oral features. Funeral ceremonies customarily include a commemorative meal profuse in food and drinks. Thereby the deceased is, in a way, incorporated into oneself by eating. Through identification the mourner frequently acquires characteristics of the deceased. For example, the son who has lost his father sometimes begins to behave like his dead father. In a person who is inclined to depression it is enough for depression to get provoked that his self-esteem is diminished as result of some disappointment or insult having harmed his self-respect.
The self-accusations of a person suffering from depression are actually self-accusations only on one level. On another level the accusations are directed to the object even though the patient is not aware of this. Anger is directed to the patient himself since through introjection he has identified himself with the lost object. Loss of the object is experienced as having become forsaken and therefore anger is roused.
There is always a grain of truth in the patient's guilt feelings. An integral part is depression is a difficulty in sustaining self-esteem high enough, which actually is always the fundamental issue in depression. Freud (1916) noticed that in depression the discharging factor is the loss of some object which is essentially important to one's self-esteem. According to psychodynamic views, the same mechanism is working both in psychotic and neurotic depression, only so that in psychoses it exists in an intensified form. The depressive person has difficulties with his own hostility. He is unable to discharge his hostility outwards without harming his personal relationships, while in the same time maintaining these relationships is very important to him in order to gain some support to his weak self-esteem. On the other hand, a person who is depressive or susceptible to depression exhibits in his close and established personal relationships very often pretentious, dependent, touchy, egocentric and pronouncedly ambivalent traits.
Bibring developed his theory of depression in 1953. In his opinion, depression is a basic reaction just like fear. Depression is a reaction to helplessness and psychic pain (Joffe and Sandler 1967). Helplessness may be real or imaginary. Psychic pain denotes various unpleasant psychic feelings, of which the most common ones include anxiety, agitation and frustration. It has been regarded generally that the separation experienced by the child in his mother-relationship has some connections with the development of depression in later years. An important area where helplessness may be experienced involves self-esteem. If the person fails to reach the ideals which have been set high, the ego experiences worthlessness which leads to development of depression. According to Bibring, aggression, which previously has been considered to be of prime importance in the origin of depression, were only of secondary nature, and the function of aggression were to alleviate anxiety in difficult situation arousing helplessness. Accordingly, aggression were

mainly a defense reaction and at the same time an attempt of restitution. Rado (1951) has described the personality of a person prone to depression, and he has paid attention to the difficulties such a person has in maintaining his self-esteem. Such a person is exceptionally vulnerable, impatient and support-seeking. His self-respect does not depend on his real achievements, but he feels comfortable only in atmosphere of warmth, love and security. It is very difficult for this kind of a person to value his own thoughts and accomplishments unless someone else supports them. Through pleasing and submission he endeavors to please others but when he has become assured of a person's love he may turn exacting and tyrannical toward his close people.

Depression is a basic reaction against psychic pain. Psychic pain is brought forth in a situation where the defence mechanisms of the ego are not capable of diverting anxiety out of consciousness.

The depressive basic reaction is characterized by retardation and rigidity which are typical of depression. This concerns one kind of freezing reaction - like Rechardt (1965) describes it - the fundamental aim of which is, one could imagine, to attenuate anxiety.

The premorbid personality of a depression-prone person is characterized by accentuated needs of dependency, very great demands made on oneself and frequently even obsessive-compulsive features. Typically, many depressive patients are careful, scrupulous, often also religious and loyal to the establishment, political party and native country. His pronounced aspiration to belong to one group or another represents his attempt to disguise his loneliness. It has already been mentioned how a depressive person often has premorbidly set his goals very high. He accomplishes his work well, he is often industrious and successful and he has a feeling that his close people need him. On the other hand, in his innermost soul he frequently feels unhappy and lonely. Often the patient has a fairly good insight into his own problems, but he is unable to solve them. Occasionally the patient is bothered by the feeling that he is not free and easy in his personal relationships but is in a way acting. In such a case he appears better externally than in his innermost, since he is plagued by the feeling that others would not appreciate him as such as he really is. The patient may be harassed by the feeling that life is void and meaningless. He frequently tends to depreciate himself.

Needs of dependency may cause a need to deny them and, on the other hand, inclination to depression and feelings of inferiority. It is usually difficult for the patients to express love actively, instead they wish to become loved. Their self-esteem is governed by external conditions. As for love affairs and relationships with friends, selection of the object may occur quite narcissistically, with the result that the patient grows attached to a person who resembles himself. The basis of all this is usually a need to maintain sufficient self-esteem. The patients change objects frequently, since time after time they disappoint in their wish for love. Depression-prone persons may exhibit obsessions and other symptoms of the obsessive-compulsive category, and such features may be noticed in their hobbies, too. They frequently deny their hostility by means of reaction formation (Fenichel 1971).

Fixation to the oral stage of psychosexual development is typical of the future depression-patient. The ego of the depressive patient endeavors to maintain peace of mind through "oral" means. Some time in the past this has been a safe stage, to which one regressively returns in depression. Many of these patients abuse alcohol, drugs or love. They may grow fat and weight changes are common. Food and drinks may symbolize security, love and warmth. It is of utmost importance to such a person to become loved, since without love life appears entirely worthless as anxiety and feelings of inferiority are straining to reach consciousness. The superego of the depressive patient is strick and frequently attacks his own ego. In order to appease his strict conscience the patient may work hard or employ masochistic measures to mitigate the accusations by the superego and the anxiety resulting from them. Often the patient's mind fluctuates between guilt feelings and more or less denied wish to make others feel guilty. Anxiety may be associated with fear of inexplicable, unconscious danger lying ahead. Depression is often connected with a previously experienced feeling of loss. Depression is usually associated with loss of a loved person, breaking of a close relationship or with experiences in work or elsewhere humiliating one's self-esteem. The common feature in all these instances is a loss in front of which the patient feels helpless.

"A woman aged forty-three years, who had previously suffered from mild temporary depressive symptoms, fell ill with a grave depression when she "lost" her only son as he married. Even though the patient on the conscious level considered it natural that children grow up and move away from home in due course of time and even though she consciously did not accept her own wish of possession, bereavement of this kind still caused grave depression".

A depression-prone person suffers from inner helplessness. Quite often he is afraid of falling under the authority of other people, if such a situation provokes feelings of helplessness in him. Such a person tends to take advantage of other people in a manipulatory way in order to acquire support and security he is longing for. If he fails in this anxiety or masked hostility may ensue even though he perhaps remains entirely unaware of this. A person who has a disposition to depression may charge other people with exorbitant demands. In order to overcome his inner uncertainty and feelings of helplessness he may submit himself into one kind of a contest (Bonime 1966). The dependency of a depression-prone person often has demanding features, too. When he gets frustrated in such demands he becomes anxious or depressed, develops psychosomatic symptoms or grows sullen. The depressive person often appears extremely dependent. He may count on others' getting concerned or behave in an appealing way. On the other hand, this attitude hampers equal and mature personal relationships and leads to feelings of loneliness. Fear of failure may bring on fear of responsibility. The aggressiveness of a depressive patient is caused by his helplessness. Aggression is an easier affect to bear than helplessness or anxiety. On the other hand depression gets directed toward oneself since expressing aggression outwards may harm personal contacts and preclude acquisition of the security which is absolutely necessary to the depression-prone person for maintenance of his self-esteem. Through his symptoms the depressive person may bring suffering upon others and thereby discharge his aggressive emotions. There is often a grain of truth in the guilt feelings. According to Bonime (1966), grave guilt feelings always include manipulative elements. When one brings forth plenty enough of his guilt and wortlessness, other people begin to believe that there are not sufficient grounds for those guilt feelings. Often the patient himself suffers extremely intensively.
In the childhood of a depressive patient there have often occurred neglecting, rejection or reactive oversolicitude by the parents. In order to cope with the situation he had had to work up his character in the described fashion, and this arrangement is repeated in other personal relationships throughout his life. A person disposed to depression suffers from feelings of inner emptiness. Guilt feelings and a strick superego may evoke masochistic features and a negative therapeutic reaction. Depressive patients seek security and approving in various ways.

Differential diagnosis

Sometimes it may prove difficult to differentiate between psychotic depression and depression of neurotic degree. Psychotic depression is characterized by a disturbance in the sense of reality, severity of self-accusations and motor inhibition. Moreover there may occur even delusions in psychotic depression. In psychotic depression the risk of suicide is greater than in neurotic depression, and in such cases it is justified to consider to admit the patient into hospital treatment. In psychotic depressions irrelistic self-accusations are strikingly clear. In psychotic depression the patient often wakes up in the early hours of the night in an agitated state and is unable to fall asleep any more. The morning and fo-

renoon are usually the most difficult times of the day in depression. Occasionally difficulties arise in the case of schizophrenic and schizo-affective psychoses which bear depressive traits. Most often there are no auditory hallucinations at all in depressive and manic psychoses. Such hallucinations would rather suggest a schizophrenic or schizo-affective psychosis. A disorder belonging to the category of manic-depressive psychosis is of a period character. Personality, is not disintegrated in the same way as in schizophrenia. Hallucinations and delusions are not typical symptoms, but the patient may exhibit paranoid features as well as rich use of projection as a defence mechanism against anxiety. The last mentioned traits approach symptoms which are met with in paranoid psychoses. In depressive psychoses the paranoid symptoms lie, however, more in the background only, and instead the depressive affective disturbance is the foremost manifestation. Stuporous states most frequently indicate catatonia, but occasionally, even if rarely, depression may manifest itself in the form of stupor.
Reactive psychoses may include either manic or depressive features, but in these cases external psychogenic factors are conspicuous and obvious. It is worth paying attention to those remarks which were mentioned earlier in this presentation about the diagnostic aspects of reactive psychoses in general.

REFERENCES

Abraham, K. (1911). Notes on the Psychoanalytical Investigation and Treatment of Manic-Depressive Insanity and Allied Conditions. In: Selected Papers on Psychoanalysis. Basic Books, New York 1953.
Achté, K., E. Hillbom and V. Aalberg (1967). Post-Traumatic Psychoses Following War Brain Injuries. Reports from the Rehabilitation Institute for Brain-Injured Veterans, I.
Angst, J. (1966). Zur Ätiologie und Nosologie endogener depressiver Psychosen. Monogr. Gesamtgeb. Neurol. Psychiat., Heft 112, Springer Verlag, Berlin.
Angst, J., and P. Weiss (1968). Ätiologie und Verlauf endogener Depressionen. In F. Labhardt (Ed.), Depressionen und ihre Behandlung, S. Karger, Basel.
Bibring, E. (1953). The Mechanisms of Depression. In P. Greenacre (Ed.)., Affective Disorders, International Universities Press, New York.
Bonime, W. (1966). The Psychodynamics of Neurotic Depression. In S. Arieti (Ed.), American Handbook of Psychiatry, Vol. III. Basic Books, New York.
Fenichel, O. (1971). The Psychoanalytic Theory of Neurosis. Routledge and Kegan Paul Ltd., London.
Freud, S. (1916). Trauer und Melancholie. Ges. Werke X. S. Fischer-Verlag, Frankfurt am Main 1963.
Grinker, R.R., J. Miller, M. Sabshin, R. Nunn and J.C. Nunnally (1961). The Phenomena of Depressions. Hoeber Medical Division, Harper and Row, New York.
Joffe, W.G. and J. Sandler (1967). On the Concept of Pain, with Special Reference to Depression and Psychogenic Pain. J. Psychosom. Res., 11, 69-75.
Kendell, R.E. (1968). Classification of Depressive Illness. Oxford University Press, London.
Ottoson, J.O. (1969). Depressionstillstandens nosologi. In: Depressiosymposium. Merck, Helsinki.
Perris, C. (1966). A study of Bipolar (Manic-Depressive) and Unipolar Recurrent Depressive Psychoses. Acta Psychiat. Scand., Suppl. 194.
Rado, S. (1951) Psychodynamics of Depression from the Etiologic Point of View. Psychosom. Med. 13, 51-55.
Rechardt, E. (1965). Neuroottiset depressiot. Duodecim 81, 361-363.
Spitz, R. (1946). Anaclitic Depression. The Psychoanalytic Study of the Child 2, 313-342.

Hostility in Depression

G. C. Lyketsos

Athens University Department of Psychiatry, Dromokaition Hospital, Athens, Greece

ABSTRACT

In recent studies it was found that cognitive changes of hostility precede affective changes in melancholia. General bipolar (extra and intropunitive) hostility scored highly. Intropunitive hostility followed in particularly high values. Similar sequence of hostility was found in the melancholic Ajax as described by Sophocles in the homonymous ancient greek drama.

KEY WORDS

Depression, Hostility, changes, ancient tragedy

INTRODUCTION

The vicsissitudes of hostility in mania and depression were known to the ancient Greeks. According to the myth: Ajax, the Telamonius, was taken by mania when the glorious weapons of the dead Achilles were casted to honour Ulysses rather than himself. Blinded by his rage, he took vengeance by killing Ulysses's sheep which he mistook to be his soldiers and the ram believing that he was killing his hated opponent.
When Ajax discovered his mistake, he felt his self-esteem degraded and deeply depressed, turning his hostility against himself committed suicide.
Homer recited Ajax's hostility by the words of Ulysses to the spirit of the dead Ajax as follows: "Aias, son of peerless Telamon, wast thou then not even in death to forget they whrath against me because of those accursed arms?".
Sophocles' powerful language speaks of the sequence of Ajax's hostilities, when he sunk into his depression as follows:
Zeus father of my fathers
How can I strike them down
that devious, hateful rogue and the two joined kings
and last find death myself?
(Straight forward expression of hostility against the depriving kings).

And now Ajax - what is to be done now?
I am hated by the gods, that's plain; the Greek camp hates me.
Troy and the ground I stand upon detest me.
(Projection of hostility towards others: Lowering of self esteem. Depressed ideas).
Shall I make a rush against the walls of Troy?
Join with them all in single combat, to
some notable exploit, and find my death in it?
Let a man nobly live or nobly die.
Go swift and punishing Erinues (1.842) (Introjection of hostility, Suicidal ideas.
Efforts to recover self esteem).
And Ajax falls onto his sword and collapses behind the bushes.
The psychodynamics of hostility in depression were explicitly analysed since the early years of the 20th century. Freud as early as 1897 mentioned hostility in depression but in 1917 he spoke of introjection, a concept that the took over from Ferenczi,as an unconscious introjective mechanism, which prevailing in depressed patients turns hostility against the self.
Mechanisms of projection of hostility against others were also observed in function amongst depressed patients (Abraham I911, 1916, Freud 1917, Lewis 1934).
According to the psychodynamic hypothesis an early depressive process is established in childhood. Then unconscious introjection conceals hostility and punitiveness against a disapointing or lost object. This introjection supports repression and denial and thereby control of the feared and disowned hostile drives.
During adulthood a significant loss may trigger a regressive repetition of the prototype or a modified depressive process. This is characterized by defusion of the object into libidinal and aggressive destructive cathexes associated with ambivalent feeling towards it. Unconcsious introjection and indentification with the negative aspects of the object follows associated with negative feelings of guilt and despair. The endogain is that the external object is saved from the accumulated defused hostility, retains its positive aspects and thus it is recovered in the phantasy of the depressed patient.
Melanie Klein claimed introjection-projection mechanisms as a process inseparable from the organisms' perceptional (or intake) and discharge system. This basic psychological commerce with the external world or object relationship begins soon after birth.
An object in the Freudian sense is that of an emotional drive. The first of these is the mother's breast, a "part object". The infant incorporates it as a "good object" but in the context of frustration having projected on to the breast his own rage he incorporates a "bad object"also. These are the prime instances of projection and introjection mechanisms that persist throughout life.
The "depressive position" as described by Melanie Klein is reached by the infant when he recognizes his mother as a real whole object both good and bad. But this new constellation ushers into a depressive anxiety situation. The infant at that stage is still under the way of uncontrollable hostile impulses. Thus fear predominates that of destruction and the loss of the loved object in the external world and in his own inside. Gradually the depressive phantasies give rise to the wish to repair and restore and in successful development the experience of love from the environment slowly reassures the infant about his objects.
Several authors argue that hostility is secondary to other primary factors. As such Balint consideredthe deep narcissistic trauma due to the loss of the archaic preambivalent love of the object, Bibring the "ego's shocking awareness of its helplessness in regard to its aspiration..." followed by precipitation of self esteem. Zetzel the inability of passive tolerance of helplessness and Hill the catastrophic lowering of self esteem.
However, a fair amount of objective evidence has now been accumulated showing the cardinal role of hostility, in particular hostility directed inwards, in depressive illness, though this evidence does not assign an aetiological role to hostility.
Recently several researchers (Mayo 1967; Philip 1971; Blackburn 1974) have found

Fould's hostility and Direction of Hostility Questionnaire (HDHQ) (Foulds et al. 1960, Foulds 1965) a useful instrument for studying the various aspects of aggression in depressive illness. The questionnaire is made up of 51 items from the MMPI and uses Rosenweig's (1934) terms, intro - and extrapunitiveness to define the bipolar direction of hostility.
In a recent study of Greek depressed patients under treatment we found, with Blackburn, that the pattern of change in hostility with recovery from depression agrees with previous results (Mayo 1967, Philip 1971, Blackburn 1974): general hostility decreases: in particular, hostility directed towards the self and a balance becomes established between intropunitiveness and extrapunitiveness. The results of this study supported the finding that extrapunitiveness tends to be stable from depression to recovery.
Although only a small number of subjects were included, this study extends the validity of Hostility and Direction of Hostility Questionnaire (HDHQ) by replicating previous findings in a sample of severely depressed patients from a different sub-culture. It seems that severe depressive illness expresses itself in a similar way cross-nationally in a high level of general hostility and over predominance of intropunitiveness.
Another problem which occupied us was the temporal relationship between hostility and depressed mood.
In a cognitive theory A.T.Beck (1967, 1972, 1976) argued that the main deficit of depression is the primary negative cognitive triad i.e. the negative view of self, of the present and the future. All other symptoms, whether affective or motivational, are secondary to the primary cognitive defect. We decided to test out Beck's theory with regard to hostility.
Since intro- and extrapunitiveness (as tested by the HDHQ) can be seen as examples of negative views of self and others, it was hypothesized that changes in hostility should precede changes in mood i.e. and individual first views himself as unworthy, bad, incopetent etc, then feels depressed. Conversely, therefore, during treatment these cognitive modes will change before a change of mood occurs.
In this study the hypothesis that changes in mood follow changes in cognitive measures of hostility was not sufficiently supported by the Beck and Hamilton questionnaires. However, there was an above chance tendency in intropunitiveness and Direction of Hostility to precede changes in mood. Nurses' ratings supported the hypothesis at a statistically significant level: Intropunitiveness and direction of hostility predicted depressed mood and anxiety.
The results provided enough encouragement to pursue this line of study further but is must be stressed that establishing the temporal precedence of hostility to mood does not imply a one to one causal relationship.
Another problem is the cultural influence in hostility and depression. Kendell (1970) looked at the relationship between hostility and depression from an epidemiological point of view and found that there tends to be an inverse relationship between suicide and homicide, that subcultures which discourage outward expressions of aggression (e.g. middle European Jews) have a higher depression rate, that depression is uncommon in pre-literate societies, that women are more prone to depression than men and older men more so than younger men. This epidemiological evidence supports the hypothesis that depression is caused by the frustration of the aggressive response but, as Kendell points out, these types of study are beset with methological pitfalls.
In a more recent study with Blackburn, we tried to elucidate the relationship between the dysthymic symptoms of depression and anxiety and hostility personality traits namely extrapunitiveness, intropunitiveness and dominance in the general Greek population, and to compare the results with the British samples. We used the lately developed tests by Foulds, the SAD for the symptoms of anxiety and depression together, and the Personality Deviance Scale (PDS).
We found a sizeable difference between the scores of depression and anxiety together obtained by the British sample and those of the total Greek sample ($P < 0.001$). At the same time the Greeks were significantly more extrapunitive

and dominant than the British (P < 0.5 and P < 0.001) and the British sample was more intropunitive than the Greek sample at a very high level of significance (P < 0.001).
The personality differences which we found in intropunitiveness, extrapunitiveness and dominance between the Greek and the British samples reflect national characteristics which may appear to have prima facie validity by confroming to national stereotypes. The lover level of intropunitiveness and higher levels of extrapuntiveness and dominance in the Greeks, as compared with the British, may give more indication why the Greek may cope better with more symptoms of depression and anxiety than his British counterpart.
According to Foulds and Bedford (1977c), high intropunitive scores increase the likelihood of developing symptoms, while high extrapunitive scores decrease the likelihood of symptoms leading to break down. It may be that their relatively high level of extrapuntiveness and dominace and lower intropunitiveness give the Greeks more protection against the development of symptoms of depression and anxiety and psychic breakdown.
In conclusion, the changes of hostility in depression are complex.
Some evidence arises from recent pieces of research:
1. In psychotic depression, general hostility and particurarly its self punitive part, score highly as measured by Fould's HDHQ. During treatment these scores decrease first and then they are followed by the clinical improvement and the improvement of depressed feelings.
2. Differences in intra-exgrapunitiveness and dominance as hostility traits seem to influence disability due to dysthymic states in the general population.
Other studies in progress give evidence that a high score of self-punitiveness as measured by the HDHQ is not exclusive in depression. It was found high in patients suffering from another major non organic psychiatric illness though not as high as in depressed patients. Moreover, low scores of dominance, a hostile personality trait, as measured by Fould's Personality Deviance Scale were found in patients who manifested physical expressions of psychopathology.

REFERENCES

Abraham, K. (1911). Notes on the psychoanalytic investigations and treatment of manic depressive insanity and allied conditions. In Selected Papers in Psychoanalysis (ed) Basic Books: New York 1960.
Abraham K. (1916). The first pregenital stage of the libido. Selected Papers in Psychoanalysis (ed) Basic Books New York 1960.
Balint M. (1952). New beginnings and the paranoid and the depressive syndromes, Int. J. Psych. anal. 33:214-23.
Beck A.T. (1976). Cognitive Therapy and Emoticnal Disorders New York. International Universities Press.
Bibring E. (1953). The mechanism of depression in affective disorders. Int. Univ. Press. pp: 13-48.
Blackburn I.M. (1974). The pattern of hostility in affective illness. British Journal of Psychiatry 125, 141-145.
Blackburn I.M., Lyketsos G.C. and Tsiantis John (1979). The temporal relatinoship between hostility and depressed mood. British J. of Social and Clinical Psychology 18, 227-235.
Foulds G.A., Caine T.M. and Creasy M.A. (1960). Aspects of extra-and intropunitive expression in mental illness. Journal of Mental Science 106, 599-6I0.
Foulds G.A. (1965). Personality and Personal Illness. Tavistock: London.
Foulds G.A. (1976). The Hierarchical Nature of Personal Illness. Academic Press: London.

Foulds G.A. and Bedford A. (1977a). Hierarchies of personality deviance and personal illness. British J. of Medical Psychology 50, 73-78.
Freud S. (1897). It is reported by Prof. Kouretas in "Eccentric characters in ancient drama".
Freud S. (1917). Mourning and Melancholia. In Collected Papers (ed) Hogarth Press London 1950.
Hill Sir Denis (1968). Depression: disease, reaction, or posture? American Journal of Psychiatry 125, 445-457.
Kendell R.F. (1970). Relationship between aggression and depression. Archives of General Psychiatry 22, 308-318.
Klein M. (1935). A contribution to the psychogenesis of manic-depressive states. Contributions to Psychoanalysis. London, Hogarth Press 1948: 282-310.
Kouretas D. (1951). Abnormal characters in Greek Ancient Drama. Edition Papanikolaou (In Greek).
Lewis A.J. (1934). Melancholia: a clinical survey of depressive states. Journal of Mental Science 80, 329-378.
Lykas D. (1972). Aias Sofocleous (Ancient text, Introduction, translation and notes). Papiros (In Greek).
Lyketsos G.C., Ivy M. Blackburn, and Tsiantis J.(1976). The movement of hostility during recovery from depression. Psychological Medicine I, 777-777.
Lyketsos G.C., Blackburn Ivy M., Mouzaki D. (1979). Personality variables and dysthymic symptoms: a comparison between a Greek and a British sample. Psychological Medicine 9, 753-758.
Mayo P.R. (1967). Some psychological changes associated with improvement in depression. British Journal of social and Clinical Psychology 6, 63-68.
Philip A.E. (1971). Psychometric changes associated with response to drug treatment. British Journal of social and Clinical Psychology. 10, 138-143.
Rosenweig S. (1934). Types of reaction to frustration. Journal of Abnormal and Social Psychology 29, 298-300.
Zetzel E.R. (1965). The depressive position. In P. Greenacre(ed).Affective disorders. New York Int. Univ. Press.-

The Role of Aggression in Affective Disorders and Its Relationship to Anxiety

A. Liakos, M. Markidis, A. Kokkevi, G. Trikkas, G. Tambouratzis and C. Stefanis

Department of Psychiatry, University of Athens, Eginition Hospital, Athens, Greece

ABSTRACT

The relationship of anxiety to aggression in neurosis and psychotic depression seems to be rather complex. Introverted Hostility is recognised as a significant factor in depression. This same factor and self criticism in particular are also strongly related to anxiety in both neurotic and psychotic depression. Aggression is a complex concept and Introverted Hostility and Intrapunitive Reactions to Frustration do not follow the same direction of relationships to anxiety in neurosis. Impunitive Responses to Frustration are negatively related to anxiety in psychotic depression. Depressive symptomatology is related to some Hostility variables while the diagnostic signs of psychotic depression are not related to aggression or anxiety.

KEYWORDS

Neurosis; psychotic depression; agression; anxiety.

INTRODUCTION

The role of aggression in affective disorders is traditionally based on psychodynamic theories and clinical observation. Abraham (1927) first considered aggression as aetiologically significant in depression. Freud (1922) in an attempt to interpret the self destructive phenomena in depression postulated the existence of a destructive instinct and considered depression as the result of internalised aggression originally addressed to a lost love object. Klein (1934) considers the predisposition to depression to be related to predominance of hostile feelings towards the integrated mother object. Other dynamic formulations consider depression a result of inhibition of the expression of aggression (Davies, 1957; Kendel, 1970).

Psychodynamic formulations however are not readily subjected to empirical objective validation. Attempts towards this direction thus far support some of the Kleinian formulations and the inhibition of aggression theory (Cochrane, 1975; Pilowsky and Spence, 1975). Methodological problems, related to the complex theoretical concepts of aggression and the diagnosis of depression, may partly be responsible for the difficulties with empirical validation studies. Objective measurement of aggression and its components is not very satisfactory and the controversy about the classification of affective disorders is still persisting and mainly centered on the validity of distinction between neurotic and psychotic depression.

Various theoretical formulations exist about the nature of aggression, deriving from psychoanalytic, ethological, psychological and social learning theories. Hostility, defined as an inherent tendency to commit an aggressive act has been measured in a number of studies for elucidating the significance of aggression in affective disorders. The concept of internal or external direction of hostility has been mainly employed and, as measuring instruments, the Fould's Hostility and Direction of Hostility Questionnaire and the Rosenzweig's Picture Frustration Test which is compatible to the frustration-aggression hypothesis of aggression, have been used. Anger as an emotional component of aggressive behaviour has also been the subject of attention in some studies. There are several investigations of the role of hostility in affective disorder, using the Fould's H.D.H.Q. Mayo (1967) tested a mixed group of neurotic and psychotic depressives before and after improvement and found a significant drop in Intrapunitive Hostility and no significant change in Extrapunitive Hostility. Philip (1971) also found a significant difference in Intrapunitive Hostility between improved and nonimproved depressives and Blackburn (1974), tested manic patients and unipolar and bipolar depressives. She found that manic patients were more Extrapunitive, while the two groups of unipolar and bipolar depressives were more Intrapunitive. Similar results were also obtained by other authors in Greece using the Fould's H.D.H.Q. (Lyketsos et al, 1976).

The conclusions from these studies support the notion that Intrapunitive Hostility and depression are related.

Pilowsky and Spence (1975) however investigated the importance of self reported Anger in psychotic and nonpsychotic depressed patients and found that the higher the psychoticism score the more likely that the patient would report Anger. This finding suggests a relationship between depression and externally directed Hostility. Furthermore, Schless and his associates (1974), in a factor analytic study on the role of hostility in depression, found that approximately half of the depressed patients showed predominance of outwardly directed hostility and Weissman and co-workers (1971) found that depressed patients directed their aggression inwards when seen by a psychiatrist, but directed it outwards when they interacted with their relatives.

In a number of studies we have investigated the relationship of aggression to anxiety, using the Fould's measures and the Rosenzweig's Picture Frustration Test. (Liakos, Markidis, Kokkevi and Stefanis,1977; Liakos, 1978;1979; Stefanis, Liakos, Kokkevi and Markidis, 1980). In both neurotic patients and psychotic depressives, we have found a significant and complex relationship between aggression and anxiety. Our results are briefly presented in the tables of this text. A strong, positive relationship, between Anxiety and Introverted Hostility in neurotics, accounting for nearly half of the variance is shown in Table 1. Self Criticism is the more

TABLE 1   Relationships of Anxiety and Hostility in 25 Neurotics

	Fould's H.D.H.Q.	A-State	A-Trait
Extroverted Hostility	Acting out Hostility	.308	.297
	Delusional "	.116	.201
	Criticism of Others	.186	.126
Introverted Hostility	Delusional Guilt	.545**	.374
	Self Criticism	.672**	.624**

Stepwise Regression Analysis
Dependent Variable: A-State

Independent Variables	Multiple R	Cumulative proportion of variance	F
Step 1 Self Criticism	.672	.452	18.96***
Step 2 Delusional Guilt	.688	.473	9.87***
Step 3 Acting out Hostility	.699	.488	6.68**

Dependent Variable A-Trait

Step 1 Self Criticism	.624	.390	14.67***
Step 2 Acting out Hostility	.638	.407	7.56**
Step 3 Criticism of Others	.653	.426	5.205*

*p < .05, **p < .01, ***p < .001

important subscale for this relationship. The same relationship but in the inverse direction exists between Anxiety and Intrapunitive Responses to Frustration as measured by the Rosenzweig P-F Test accounting for roughly one third of the variance (Liakos et al., 1977). This would at first appear contradictory. It

TABLE 2 Relationships of Anxiety and Reactions to Frustration in 25 Neurotics

Rosenzweig's P-F test	A-State	A-Trait
Extrapunitive Response	.209	.386
Intrapunitive "	-.467*	-.572**
Impunitive "	.123	-.028
Object Dominance	-.179	-.239
Group Conformity Response	.116	.423*

Stepwise Regression Analysis
Dependent Variable: A-State

Independent Variables	Multiple R	Cumulative proportion of variance	F
Step 1 Intrapunitive Response	.467	.218	6.42**
Step 2 Object Dominance	.523	.274	4.15*
Step 3 Group Conformity Response	.532	.283	2.76

Dependent Variable: A-Trait

Step 1 Intrapunitive Response	.572	.327	11.19***
Step 2 Group Conformity Response	.749	.561	14.07***
Step 3 Extrapunitive Response	.754	.569	9.24*

*p < .05, **p < .01, ***p < .001

means however that Anxiety in neurotics is linked with Self Criticism and at the same time, that Anxiety is inversely related to Intrapunitive Response to Frustration.

In Tables 3 and 4 the results of a second study showing the same relations, in psychotic depressives are presented (Liakos, 1979, Stefanis et al.,1980).

TABLE 3 Relationships of Anxiety and Hostility in 22 Psychotic Depressions

Fould's H.D.H.Q.		A-State	A-Trait
Extraverted Hostility	Acting out Hostility	.010	.053
	Delusional Hostility	-.093	.050
	Criticism of Others	-.130	.069
Introverted Hostility	Delusional Guilt	.315	.515**
	Self Criticism	.603**	.701***

Stepwise Regression Analysis
Dependent Variable: A-State

Independent Variables	Multiple R	Cumulative proportion of variance	F
Step 1 Self Criticism	.603	.364	11.43**
Step 2 Criticism of Others	.727	.529	10.65***
Step 3 Delusional Guilt	.753	.567	7.84**

Dependent Variable: A-Trait

Step 1 Self Criticism	.701	.492	19.38**
Step 2 Acting out Hostility	.758	.574	12.82***
Step 3 Criticism of others	.763	.582	8.37**

**p < .01, ***p < .001

TABLE 4 Relationships of Anxiety and Reactions to Frustration in 22 Psychotic Depressions

Rosenzweig's P-F Test	A-State	A-Trait
Extrapunitive Response	.427*	.252
Intrapunitive Response	.105	.130
Impunitive Response	-.440*	-.228

Stepwise Regression Analysis
Dependent Variable A-State

Independent Variables	Multiple R	Cumulative proportion of variance	F
Step 1 Impunitive Response	.440	.194	4.806*
Step 2 Extrapunitive Response	.465	.216	2.615

*p < .05

TABLE 7   The Interater Reliability of the Diagnostic Index and the
Hamilton Rating Scale in 22 Psychotic Depressions

	Hamilton's Scale			Diagnostic Index		
	M	S.D.	R	M	S.D.	R
Rater 1	32.18	(5.92)		9.23	(1.92)	
			0.677***			0.579**
Rater 2	33.09	(7.51)		8.32	(1.55)	

**p < .01, ***p < .001

The mean score of the two raters for the diagnostic index is well above the accepted limit of 6, for the diagnosis of psychotic depression. Table 8 shows the relationship of Hostility to the degree of depression as measured by the Hamilton rating scale.

TABLE 8   The Relationships of Hostility to the Diagnosis of Depression
and Depressive Symptomatology in 22 Psychotic Depressions

Stepwise Regression Analysis
Dependent Variable: Hamilton's Rating Scale Score

Independent Variables Fould's H.D.H.Q. Subscales	Multiple R	Cumulative Proportion of Variance	F
Step 1 Acting out Hostility	.307	.094	1.087
Step 2 Self Criticism	.526	.276	3.630*
Step 3 Criticism of Others	.581	.337	3.052
Step 4 Delusional Guilt	.595	.355	2.335
Step 5 Delusional Hostility	.608	.370	1.878

Dependent Variable: The Diagnostic Index Score
(Carney Roth and Garside)

Step 1 Delusional Hostility	.360	.129	2.975
Step 2 Acting out Hostility	.467	.218	2.652
Step 3 Delusional Guilt	.504	.254	2.039

*p < .05

A significant relationship appears with the addition of the Self Criticism subscale to Acting out Hostility, accounting for one fourth of the variance. There is no significant relationship between the Diagnostic Index score and Hostility. Table 9 shows the same analysis of the relationships between the Hamilton Rating Scale score and the Diagnostic Index score, to the Reaction to Frustration subscales. There are no significant relationships.

TABLE 9   The Relationships of the Diagnosis and the Degree of
Depression to the Reactions to Frustration in 22
Psychotic Depressions

Stepwise Regression Analysis
Dependent Variable: Hamilton's Rating Scale Score

Independent Variables Rosenzweig's P-F Test Subscales		Cumulative Proportion of Variance	F
Step 1 Group Conformity Response	.178	.032	.654
Step 2 Extrapunitive Response	.259	.067	.683

Dependent Variable: The Diagnostic Index Score
(Carney Roth and Garside)

Step 1 Group Conformity Response	.185	.034	.709
Step 2 Impunitive Response	.229	.052	.525

It is apparent from reviewing the results of other studies as well as from our own investigations that the hypothesis of a simple straightforward relationship of aggression and depressive disorders cannot be substantiated at the moment. Introverted Hostility as measured by the H.D.H.Q. appears to be a significant factor in depression. This same factor, and Self Criticism in particular, also seems to be strongly related to anxiety, an important emotion in both neurotic and psychotic depression. Aggression is not a simple concept and Introverted Hostility and Intrapunitive Reaction to Frustration do not follow the same pattern of relationships to anxiety in neurosis, the former showing a positive and the latter a negative relationship. Anxiety is also inversely related to Impunitive Responses to Frustration in psychotic depression. Depressive symptomatology as measured by the Hamilton Scale is related to Hostility and especially to its Self Criticism component, while it is not related to Reactions to Frustration. The first finding, would appear to be in accordance with classical formulations of the psychodynamics of depression and clinical observation linking depression with guilt and self depreciation. Some of the above relationships are too complex to be explained by a single theory.

The same positive and strong relationship exists between Introverted Hostility and Anxiety. This relationship with the addition of the Extroverted Hostility variables accounts for over half of the variance. This suggests an aetiological relationship. The negative relationship of anxiety to Intrapunitive Responses, found in neurotics, is here replaced by a negative relationship, to Impunitive responses to Frustration. This relationship accounts for about one fifth of the variance.

TABLE 5 Comparison of Anxiety and Hostility Relations in Neurotics and Psychotic Depressions

Foulds H.D.H.Q.	Neurotics (N = 25) A-State	A-Trait	Psychotic Depressions (N = 22) A-State	A-Trait
Delusional Guilt	.545**	N.S.	N.S.	.515**
Introverted Hostility Self Criticism	.672**	.624**	.603**	.701***

**p < .01, ***p < .001

TABLE 6 Comparison of the Relations of Anxiety and Reactions to Frustration in Neurotics and Psychotic Depressions

Rosenzweig's P-F Test	Neurotics (N = 25) A-State	A-Trait	Depressions (N = 22) A-State	A-Trait
Extrapunitive Response	N.S.	N.S.	.427*	N.S.
Intrapunitive "	-.467*	-.572**	N.S.	N.S.
Impunitive "	N.S.	N.S.	-.440*	N.S.
Group Conformity	N.S.	.423*	N.S.	N.S.

*p < .05, **p < .01

The results showing the differences in the relationships of anxiety and aggression in neurotic and psychotic depressions are summarized in Table 5 and 6. Their significance has been discussed in detail elsewhere (Liakos, 1978). It is worth presenting in this paper some data derived from the above study, showing the relationships of aggression to the diagnosis of psychotic depression and the clinical manifestations of depression, as measured by the Hamilton rating scale. The diagnosis of psychotic depression was confirmed in this study by the use of Diagnostic Index for psychotic depression (Carney Roth and Garside, 1965). Both these scales were given by two independent raters and the interater reliability is shown in Table 7.

REFERENCES

Abraham, K. (1927). Notes on the psychoanalytic investigation and treatment of manic-depressive insanity and allied conditions. In K. Abraham, Selected papers on psychoanalysis. Hogarth, London.
Blackburn, I.M. (1974). Brit. J. Psychiat. 125, 141-145.
Carney, M.W.P., M. Roth, and R.F. Garside (1965). Brit. J. Psychiat., 111, 659.
Cochrane, N. (1975). Brit. J. Med. Psychol., 48, 113-130.
Davis, D. (1957). An introduction to psychopathology. Oxford University Press, London.
Freud,S. (1922). Beyond the pleasure principle. International Psychoanalytic Press, London.
Kendell, R.E. (1970). Arch. Gen. Psychiat., 22, 308-318.
Klein, M. (1974). A contribution to psychogenesis of manic-depressive states. In M. Klein, Contributions to psycho-analysis, 1921-1945. Hogarth, London.
Liakos, A., M. Markidis, A. Kokkevi, and C. Stefanis (1977). The relation of anxiety to hostility and frustration in neurotic patients. In C.D. Spielberger and I.G. Sarason (Eds.), Stress and anxiety, Vol. 4, Hemisphere, Washington D.C.
Liakos, A. (1978). The dynamics of anxiety and aggression in psychiatric disorders. In CD. Spielberger and I.G. Sarason (eds). Stress and Anxiety Vol. V, Hemisphere, Washington DC.
Liakos, A. (1979). The Relationships of Anxiety and Aggression in Psychotic Depression. Dissertation for Associate Professor's Thesis, Athens University Medical School, Athens, Greece.
Lyketsos, G.C., IM Blackburn and J. Tsiantis (1976). Psycholog. Med., I. 777.
Mayo, D. (1967). Brit. J. Clin. Psychol. 6, 63-68.
Pilowsky, I., N.D. Spense (1975). Arch. Gen. Psychiat. 32, 1154-1159.
Schless, A.P., J. Mendels, A. Kipperman, and C. Cochrane (1974). J. Nerv. Ment. Dis. 159, 91-100.
Stefanis, C., A. Liakos, A. Kokkevi and M. Markidis (1980). Interactional pattern of aggression, anxiety and psychotic depression. In Achtē K., V. Aalberg and J. Lönngvist (eds) 1980). Psychopathology of Depression. Proceedings of the Symposium by the Section of Clinical Psychopathology of the World Psychiatric Association 1979, Psychiatria Fennica Suplementum, Helsinki.
Weissman, M.M., G.L. Clerman, and E. Paykel (1971). Amer. of Psychiat. 128, 261-266.

The Relation of Obsessive-compulsive Phenomena to Anxiety in Depressive Patients

J. Liappas, A. D. Rabavilas and C. Stefanis

Department of Psychiatry, University of Athens, Eginition Hospital, Athens, Greece

ABSTRACT

The obsessive-compulsive symptoms and traits and the "state" and "trait" anxiety, measured by means of self-rating inventories, were correlated in a group of patients with primary depression and a group of anxiety neurotics. The results suggest that depressive patients demonstrate strong possitive trends between obsessional personality traits and "trait" anxiety, in contradistinction to neurotic patients. It is concluded that in primary depressive patients, anxiety and obsessional manifestations are based on the corresponding personality traits and consitute two cooperating and perhaps mutually recruited phenomena.

KEY WORDS

Obsessional symptoms and traits; "state" and "trait" anxiety; primany depression; anxiety neurosis.

INTRODUCTION

Data derived from various sources indicate that depressive and obsessional symptoms represent a by no means rare co-phenomenon in the everyday psychiatric practice. Thus, depression appears to be a common complication of the obsessive-compulsive neurosis (34% of the obsessional neurotics suffer from depression according to Rosenberg (1968)), while 31% of the depressive patients develop obsessional symptoms at some stage of their illness (Gittleson 1966). In parallel, Kendell and Discipio (1970) examining the records of 4.793 psychiatric patients, found that 414 of them were recorded as having both depression and obsessive-compulsive manifestations. Many views have been put forward to account for the relation of depression to obsessions. Stengel (1948) suggested that in many cases in which depressive and obsessional symptoms occur together, the former have exacerbated preexisting obsessional personality traits into symptoms.Similar views have been expressed by Gittleson (1966), while, conversely, Sargant and Slater (1950) suggested that patients without obsessional personalities do often develop both obsessions and depression.
The role played by obsessions occuring in a setting of depression has also been e-

xamined. Gittleson (1966) proposed that obsessions may have a protective effect against suicidal tendencies and Rosenberg (1968) pointed out their anxiety-reducing properties, while Vaughan (1976) in his retrospective study of 168 depressives found significant associations between anxiety, agitation and obsessions, contrary to Gittleson (1966), who did not find such associations. Taking into account that most of the above views are based on retrospective studies, the scope of this work is to investigate the relation of anxiety to obsessive-compulsive manifestations in a group pf currently depressed patients in comparison with a control group of neurotic patients.

MATERIAL AND METHODS

22 patients suffering from primary depression (11 females and 11 males, mean age 31.2 years ±7.2) were matched for age and sex with 22 patients with anxiety neurosis (mean age 30.7 years ±8.5). Depressive patients were all in an active period of their illness. Neurotic patients were also manifesting symptoms requiring psychiatric care at the time this investigation took place.
Both groups were administered the State-Trait Anxiety Inventory (S.T.A.I.) (Spielberger, Gorsuch and Lushene 1970) and the "symptom" and "trait" portions of the Leyton Obsessional Inventory (L.O.I.) (Cooper 1970). The S.T.A.I. provides different scores for "state anxiety", i.e. anxiety experienced at a particular moment, and for "trait anxiety", i.e. anxiety as a habitual tendency. The "symptom" portion of the L.O.I. gives separate scores for ten obsessional symptoms, while the "trait" portion of this inventory provides separate scores for eight different obsessional personality traits.

RESULTS

The mean scores of the inventories employed as well as the comparison between the groups tested are presented on Table 1.

TABLE 1 The Leyton Obsessional and the State-Trait Anxiety Inventories: Comparisons between groups.

	LEYTON OBSESSIONAL INVENTORY				STATE-TRAIT ANXIETY INVENTORY			
	"Symptom"		"Trait"		"State"		"Trait"	
	m	sd	m	sd	m	sd	m	sd
Depressives	26.40	6.37	14.47	4.75	50.13	10.11	51.40	7.39
Neurotics	21.45	7.14	11.30	3.48	48.00	11.18	51.00	9.40
t-test	2.42		2.52		0.66		0.15	
P<	0.02		0.02		ns		ns	

The two groups do not differ significantly on both "state" and "trait" anxiety. As far as the L.O.I. scores are concerned, the depressive patients show significantly more obsessional symptoms and traits as compared with the neurotics (P<0.02 for both). The correlations of the S.T.A.I. and L.O.I. scores are presented on Table 2

TABLE 2 Correlations of the L.O.I. with the
S.T.A.I. in depressive and neurotic patients (*=P<0.05, **=P<0.01)

LEYTON O.I. "Symptom"	STATE-TRAIT ANXIETY INVENTORY			
	State Anxiety		Trait Anxiety	
	Depressives	Neurotics	Depressives	Neurotics
Obsessive thoughts	.680***	.261	.167	.252
Checking	.311	.232	.344	.428*
Dirt and contamination	.293	.042	-.012	.342
Dangerous objects	.154	.248	.306	.331
Personal cleanliness and tidiness	-.312	.214	.063	.176
Household cleanliness and tidiness	-.053	.312	-.181	.334
Order and routine	-.092	.306	.130	.156
Repetition	.021	.197	-.174	.348
Over-conscientiousness and lack of satisfaction	.458*	.012	.146	.263
Indecision	.342	-.123	-.133	.152
"Trait"				
Hoarding	.252	-.343	.347	-.297
Cleanliness	.344	.234	.568**	.156
Meanness	-.236	-.156	.437*	.036
Irritable and morose	.107	.052	.432*	.208
Rigidity	.341	.295	.536**	.134
Health preoccupation	.106	-.018	.417	.035
Regularity	.012	-.032	.496*	.086
Punctuality	-.143	-.156	.402	.064

Regarding the relation of obsessional symptoms to "state anxiety", depressive patients show significant positive trends with respect to "obsessive thoughts" (P<0.01) and "over-conscientiousness" (P<0.05). In contrast, no such relations are demonstrated in neurotics. Regarding the relation of obsessional symptoms to "trait anxiety", neurotic patients show more positive trends, which for "checking" reach significant levels (P<0.05).
The main difference between groups is found with respect to the relation of obsessional traits to "trait anxiety". Depressive patients show significant positive trends regarding most of the obsessional traits investigated (P range from 0.05 to 0.01) in contradistinction to neurotic patients.

DISCUSSION

The results of this study indicate that the importance of the relation between anxiety and obsessive-compulsive phenomena in depressive patients rests upon personality traits rather than symptoms. The significant positive relation of "trait anxiety" to obsessional personality traits observed in the depressive group is in agreement with Lewis' views (1934). The importance of this finding appears to concern not only the significance of the relation as such, but also its stability over traits. Thus, while in the five out of the eight obsessional traits investigated the relationship to "trait anxiety" reaches significant levels, in the remaining three the trends are also strongly positive. Therefore, it could be suggested that a potent mutuality may exist between obsessions and anxiety at the personality traits level in depressive patients. A similar mutuality, although to a lesser extend, is found with regard overt symptoms as well, since highly significant correlations are found between "obsessive thoughts" and "over-conscientiousness" and "state anxiety" in this group. Therefore, it could be suggested that the positive association of traits may precipitate a similar relationship between symptoms. This indicates that in a setting of depression, obsessions do not have anxiety-reducing properties and therefore, Rachman's (1971) hypothesis concerning the sensitizing effects of ruminations on depressive patients' symptoms of anxiety is confirmed. Furthermore, this observation is compatible with Vaughan's retrospective findings with regard to anxiety and agitation being positively associated with obsessions in depressive patients. It can be concluded that anxiety and obsessional manifestations are not antagonistic phenomena in depression. On the contrary, it appears that they constitute two co-operating and perhaps mutually recruited mechanisms anchored on the corresponding personality traits. Having made this conclusion, one could go further and speculate that depressive conditions occurring late in life, such as involutional melancholia, may owe their late appearance to the depression-antagonizing co-action of such personality traits.

As far as neurotic patients are concerned, the obsessional traits are not significantly related to either "state" or "trait" anxiety, while the latter appears to be positively associated with certain obsessional symptoms, such as checking. Therefore, it can be assumed that in neurotic patients the relations between anxiety and obsession work on a different level as compared to depressive patients.

The findings of this work are subject to the limitations inherent to studies based on correlational data. However, they provide some grounds for a more specific future investigation with respect to depressive psychopathology.

REFERENCES

Cooper, J. (1970). Psychol. Med. 1, 48-64.
Gittleson, N.L. (1966). Brit. J.Psychiat. 112, 253-258.
Kendell, R., and W. Discipio (1970). Psychol. Med. 1, 65-72.
Lewis, A. (1934). J. ment. Sci. 80, 277-378.
Rachman, S. (1971). Behav. Res. and Therapy 9, 229-235.
Rosenberg, C.M. (1968). Brit.J. Psychiat. 114, 477-478.
Sargant, W. and E. Slater (1950) Proc. roy. soc. Med. 43, 1007-1010.
Spielberger, C.D., R.L. Gorsuch and R.E. Lushene (1970). Manual for the State-Trait Anxiety Inventory, Consulting Psychologists Press, Palo Alto.
Stengel, E. (1948). J. ment. Sci. 91, 166-187.
Vauchan, M. (1976). Brit. J. Psychiat. 129, 36-39.

Depression in the Institutionalized Elderly

C. Soldatos

Department of Psychiatry, University of Athens, Eginition Hospital, Athens, Greece

ABSTRACT

In a psychosocial study conducted in the Home for the Aged of Athens the occurence of depression and its psychosocial concommitants were assessed. Sixty five percent of the institutionalized elderly free of detectable organic brain syndrome were found to be depressed; their vast majority showed reactive depression. Physical incapacitation, lowered level of activity and complete lack of any income appeared to be factors contributing to the development of depression in the institutionalized elderly. Dealing with these factors through social, medical and public health measures may have preventive or therapeutic value.

KEYWORDS

Psychogeriatrics; depression; psychosocial factors; institutionalized elderly.

INTRODUCTION

Depression has been considered the most prevalent mental illness affecting the elderly; it may manifest itself in many ways and can cause serious difficulties with diagnosis (Whitehead, 1974). Reactive depression becomes more frequent in old age (Verwoerdt, 1976). A major factor in the development of reactive depression in the elderly is probably loss of physical health (Verwoerdt and Dovenhuehle, 1964; Zung, 1967 and Nowlin, 1974). The incidence of primary affective illness, also, increases with age (Rownsley, 1968) and this has been associated with an increase of MAO - levels as age advances (Nies et al., 1973). Consequently, it is of particular interest to determine the type of depression which is more prevalent among elderly depressed individuals and the factors possibly contributing to its development. The purpose of the present study is to describe depression in a population of institutionalized elderly and to investigate the relation between depression and various physical or mental health correlates as well as certain sociocultural characteristics.

MATERIAL AND METHODS

This study is based on material collected for another psychosocial project conducted in the Home for the Aged of Athens, a large philanthropic institution (Soldatos, 1969). In order to secure reliable historical information and completion of the psychological tests, certain inclusion criteria were required. The subjects had to be free of serious sensory deficiency or clinically detectable organic brain syndrome. Thus, although the total population of two boarding homes within the institution (N=100) was examined, only 60 subjects (30 males and 30 females) were included. They were living permanently in the institution and their age ranged from 65 to 95 years.

Our method of data collection was basically a number of interviews with each subject. During those interviews a detailed psychiatric evaluation was conducted for the purpose of recording any psychiatric symptoms and a series of psychological characteristics for each subject. Based on the presence of the symptom of depression the subjects were distinguished in two groups. To test the relationship between depression in the elderly and certain possible psychosocial factors for its development the group of depressed subjects was compared with the group of non-depressed individuals. Chi square analysis was employed for all comparisons, except for the comparison of the mean age for which the Student t-test was utilized. The two groups were not matched for age and sex; however these two parameters were not found to be significantly different.

RESULTS

The psychiatric evaluation revealed that depression was present in 65% of the sample (N=39), whereas anxiety in 38% (N=23) and paranoid tendencies in 10% (N=6). When comparing the two groups it was found that the sex distribution did not significantly differ between the depressed (46% male and 54% female) and the non-depressed (57% male and 43% female). The two groups, also did not significantly differ in terms of their mean age, which was 77.26 (±0.95) for the depressed and 78.67 (±1.70) for the non-depressed.

Depression, whenever present, varied in degree. Most often, however, it was relatively mild without intense depressive ideation. In only two cases with a history suggestive of manic-depressive illness, death wishes were communicated. However, none of the subjects expressed suicidal ideas. All but two of the depressed subjects presented with what is commonly called "reactive depression", but the depressive mood was seldom consciously attached to the stressful environmental conditions and / or the problems of aging. In most cases, although depression was subjectively experienced as an emotional state and its expression was evident in the patient's overall behavior, it was not associated by them to situational factors. Most of the elderly were using such ego defenses as rationalization, intellectualization and denial and they did not appear to be consciously concerned with their condition.

TABLE 1. Physical and Mental Health Correlates

	Depressed (N=39)	Non-Depressed (N=21)	x^2 test
Present Physical Status			
General Health Good	41%	57%	
Fair	59%	43%	N.S.
Functional Ability Good	51%	86%	
Fair	49%	14%	p<0.01
Activity Level Considerable	31%	67%	
Very limited	69%	33%	p<0.01
Emotional Correlates			
Feeling Rejected Yes	85%	52%	
No	15%	48%	N.S.
Self-esteem None	54%	24%	
Some	46%	76%	p<0.05
Anxiety Yes	51%	14%	
No	49%	86%	p<0.01
Paranoid Tendencies Yes	13%	5%	
No	87%	95%	N.S.

Depression was not found to be related to the subjects' general health in terms of the presence of various physical illnesses (Table 1). Nevertheless, a specific physical incapacitation in relation to limited functional ability and a lowering of the overall activity level independent from the general health status were each positively related to depression.

When several emotional correlates were considered, it was found that more depressed than non-depressed individuals were feeling rejected. However, this difference was not statistically significant. As shown in table 1, depression was significanly related to loss of self-esteem and the presence of anxiety, but not with the presence of paranoid tendencies.

TABLE 2. Sociocultural Characteristics

		Depressed (N=39)	Non-Depressed (N=21)	x^2 test
Sociocultural Background				
Native Area	Rural	36%	48%	
	Urban	64%	52%	N.S.
Education	Grade School	59%	38%	
	Higher	41%	62%	N.S.
Marital Status	Single	28%	19%	
	Other	72%	81%	N.S.
Religiosity	Strong	79%	62%	
	Weak	21%	38%	N.S.
Present Social Status				
Income	None	46%	24%	
	Some	54%	76%	$p<0.05$
Years of institunalization	One or less	41%	33%	
	More than one	59%	67%	N.S.
Number of beds in room	One or two	33%	43%	
	More than two	67%	57%	N.S.

When comparing parameters related to the psychosocial background of our subjects (native area, education, marital status and religious belief) we did not observe statistically significant differences between depressed and non-depressed individuals (Table 2). When, however, the current socioeconomic status was considered, it was found that complete lack of any income was significantly related to the presence of depression. This was not the case with the duration of stay in the institution and the type of accomodation within it.

DISCUSSION

The results of this study confirm previous reports on the high incidence of depression in the elderly (Roth, 1955 and Batchelor, 1957). In our sample of institutionalized elderly, not only the majority showed depression, but depression was by far the most prevalent psychiatric condition. The diagnosis of reactive depression was established in almost every case and several factors possibly contributing to its development were detected. Nevertheless, an increase in MAO levels and a decrease in nonepinephrine levels as age progresses may constitute a predisposing factor (Coppen, 1967 and Robinson et al., 1972), at least in some cases. In such cases, a biological vulnerability to the development of depression may constitute the substrate upon which psychosocial factors might have elicited what was clinically diagnosed as "reactive depression".
Previous studies have indicated that mental disturbances are more prevalent in groups with lower income and limited education. (Hollingshead and Redlich, 1958 and Srole et al., 1962). Our data show that depression in the aged is indeed related to lower income.
Limited education did not show a statistically significant relation to depression, but this was probably due to the relatively small sample size. Among the Paramaters of the present socioeconomic status the duration of stay in the institution and the conditions of the accomodation did not appear to be related to the presence of depression. It seems possible that the most decisive factor in the development of depression is living in the institution per se rather than the specific conditions of the institutionalization.

Our results are in general agreement with previous reports that depression in the elderly may relate to loss of physical health (Verwoerdt and Dovenhuehle, 1964; Zung, 1967 and Nowlin, 1974). We were able to specifically point to the importance of physical incapacitation and a lowered activity level. It is possible that the lowered self-esteem, which was found to be related to depression is a by-product of the lack of income and the limitations of functional activity and activily level. However, loss of self-esteem may be a manifestation rather than a causative factor of depression. Finally, the close relationship of anxiety to depression is an indication of the reactive nature of depression and points to the need of detecting depression when anxiety is present in the institutionalized elderly.

In conclusion, the complete lack of any income, the reduction of functional ability and the lowering of activity level in the institutionalized elderly were found to be factors clearly related to the presence of depression. Dealing with these factors through social, medical and public health measures might act preventively and therapeutically to the development of depression.

REFERENCES

Batchelor, I.R.C. (1957). Suicide in old age. In Clues to Suicide, Schneidman E.S. and Farberow M.L. (eds) Mc Graw-Hill, New York, pp. 143-151.
Coppen, A. (1967). Br. J. Psychiat. 113, 1237-1264.
Hollingshead A., and R.C. Redlich (1958). Social class and mental illness. John Wiley and Sons. New York.
Nies A., D.S. Robinson, J.M. Davis, and C.L. Ravaris (1973). Changes is monoamine oxidase with aging. In Advances in Behavioral Biology, Vol.6, Psychopharmacology and Aging, Eisdorfer C. and W.E. Fann (eds). Plenum Press, New York, pp 41-54.
Nowlin, J.B. (1974). Depression and health. In Normal aging, Vol. 2, Palmore E. (Ed.) Duke University Press, Durham N.C. pp. 168-172.
Robinson D.S., A. Nies, J.N. Davis, W.E. Bunney, J.M. Davis, R.W. Colburn, H.R. Bourne, D.M. Shaw, and A.J. Coppen (1972). Lancet 1, 290-291.
Roth M. (1955). J. Ment. Sci. 101, 281-301.
Rownsley K. (1968). Br. J. Psychiat. (special publication No 2) 27-36.
Soldatos, C. (1969). Death as a psychological problem of the aged. Adamantides' Publications, Athens, Greece.
Srole L., T.S. Langner, S.T. Michael, M.K. Opler, T.A.C. Rennie (1962). Mental health in the metropolis: The midtown Manhattan study. Mc Graw-Hill Book Co. New York.
Verwoerdt A. (1976).Clinical Geropsychiatry. Williams and Wilkins Co. Baltimore Md.
Verwoerdt A. and R.H. Dovenhuehle (1964). Geriatrics 19, 856864.
Whitehead J.M. (1974).Psychiatric disorders in old age. Harvey Miller and Medcalf. Aylesbury, England.
Zung W.W.K. (1967). Psychosomatics 8, 287-292.

3. Psychological and Epidemiological
Aspects of Depression

Psychometric Aspects of the Depressions

M. Hamilton

Department of Psychiatry, University of Leeds, Leeds, UK

ABSTRACT

On the basis of psychometric theory, psychiatric symptoms can be quantified and thus made amenable to forms of analysis not otherwise possible. It has been shown that the clinical picture presented by patients differs in many respects, though not all, from traditional descriptions. Initial and Delayed Insomnia are not related to the pattern of symptoms. The frequency distributions of scores does not provide evidence for differences between types of depressions.

KEYWORDS

Psychometry; Hamilton Rating Scale; primary depressive illness; differences between sexes.

INTRODUCTION

It is a common belief that research in the field of medicine now always requires the use of laboratory facilities and equipment, and this is considered to apply even to psychiatry. Like many popular beliefs this one is only partly true. Clinical research can require elaborate equipment but also it can often be carried out with the minimum of tools and frequently with no more than pencil and paper. There is still room for fundamental work on the clinical phenomena of mental disorders, work which is not only of theoretical significance but also of great practical importance. The traditional descriptions of clinical syndromes are based on work carried out a long time ago on the type of patients then admitted to mental hospitals. With the development of psychiatric facilities, clinicians now see many patients who present symptoms which are much milder than those which require admission to hospital. Furthermore, the increasing acceptability of psychiatric illness and treatment by our patients means that they come for treatment at a much earlier stage of illness are not the same. For these reasons, clinicians should continually look at the phenomena which concern them. They can do this by the traditional way of observation and description, but in the last few decades they have had made available to them those quantitative techniques based on psychometric theory, which can offer new insights.
This paper is concerned with the symptomatology of depressive illness based on the data recorded on a rating scale (Hamilton 1967). A previous report given at the

World Psychiatric Association meeting held in Helskinki in 1979 was concerned largely with the findings from male patients; this paper will deal chiefly with the findings in female patients.
For this work to have any meaning, it is necessary to describe how the patients were selected, but before this a few definitions will be particularly helpful. The word "depression" is used with three different meanings and discussions on the subject are often confused by a lack of understanding of what is meant. Depression is a particular mood associated with the reaction to a loss. We become depressed when a friend or relative dies, or when we lose a job of work. It is a reaction also to a potential loss or the absence of an expected gain, e.g. when we do not get a promotion we had expected or we fail in an examination. Such depression is a normal human reaction and is recognised as such. It is clearly related to the events which have produced it, not only in time but also in intensity: a great loss makes us very depressed and a minor loss produces only a slight reaction.
We use the word depression also to describe a pathological mood. In general we distinguish most simply between normal and abnormal depressed mood, because the latter will be unrelated to external events, or be out of proportion to them. Morbid depressed mood is accompanied by other changes which indicate its nature. Thus the patients will feel that everything is worthless, that their life has been pointless, that the future is hopeless and that they will never recover. In other words, their thinking and judgement are disturbed. Some patients, who are sufficiently intelligent and capable of expressing themselves, will say that the abnormal mood is clearly distinguishable from misery and unhappiness. In what way this is so, they cannot explain in a manner which can be understood, because our comprehension of the moods and feelings of others depends on our ability to recognize the similarity between our own experience and what they are indicating by words and behaviour. A pathologically depressed mood will also be accompanied by other symptoms. It is true that it is not always easy to distinguish between normal and abnormal depression, but that does not signify that there is not fundamental difference between them or that there is no point in making the distinction. An analogy will help to make the point clearer. In the spectrum we can distinguish between the two colours green and blue, but there is a point between them where it cannot be said that the colour is definitely green or blue. That does not signify that there is no real difference between these two colours or that there is no point in trying to distinguish between them.
Depression is also used to signify a syndrome, a collection of symptoms which form a coherent pattern. This is what is sometimes called a depressive illness and is one which has a clear course, which usually is recurrent and has clear intervals between each phase, is known to have a genetic component and for which there is good evidence of an underlying biochemical disturbance.
The patients studied have all been diagnosed as suffering from a primary depressive illness, though a few are secondary to physical disease such as influenza or diabetes mellitus. In none of the patients did the symptoms appear in the course of schizophrenia, of hysterical or obsessional states. In particular, patients diagnosed as suffering from "schizo-affective" disorders were excluded. Within this group special mention must be made of the condition sometimes known as "paraphrenia", in which the patient experiences vivid auditory hallucinations but without deterioration of personality and usually accompanied by severe symptoms of depression. The last may dominate the clinical picture and the hallucinations may appear only at a later stage of the illness or when the depressive symptoms improve, perhaps as a result of treatment. Although the patient may present at first as a case of depressive illness, often there may be some anomalous symptoms, revealed by careful anamnesis, which will make the psychiatrist cautious about committing himself to a diagnosis. "Paraphrenia" should be regarded as a form of schizophrenia appearing in middle age.
One condition excluded is that which might be called "excessive depressive reaction". There is a type of emotional person who reacts excessively to circumstances. When things go well with them they are full of the joy of life, but when

things go wrong they fall into the depths of despair. Nowadays, they then come to the psychiatrist. It is important to recognise that these persons are not "ill", even though they have come to the clinic as "patients". The loss they have experienced may seem trivial, but it is important to them, and their reaction to it is consonant with their personality. Psychiatrists tend to dislike such "patients", because so often they are importunate, and they use various denigratory terms to describe them, the most innocuous of which is "emotionally labile personality". We recognize that they are not ill because their condition is firmly linked to their circumstances. If the loss is replaced or restitution occurs, then immediately all is well with such persons. The tears are replaced by smiles, the despair by hope, the suicidal thoughts by the joy of life. Because we do not regard these persons as being "ill", this does not mean that we refuse to give them such help as we can. They need comfort, reassurance and help with their problems. It is my opinion that they do not need drugs.
The figures in this report are derived from samples of 93 male (mean age about 51 years) and 110 or, for some, 75 female patients (mean age about 45 years). Most of the patients were untreated when first seen, but a few had received either antidepressive drugs for less than a week, or inadequate doses, e.g. 10mg of a tricyclic twice daily, for a longer period.

COMPARISON BETWEEN MALES AND FEMALES

It is the tradition that the three typical symptoms of depressive illness (melancholia) are Depressed Mood, Guilt and Suicide. But what is meant by "typical"? A distinction has to be made between what is most common and what is characteristic, in the sense of making the diagnosis of depressive illness very probable, and other diagnoses very improbable. The clinician who concentrates his attention on the "characteristic" symptoms is then going to miss the diagnosis quite frequently. The three commonest symptoms, both for males and females, in this series were Depressed Mood, which occured in 100% of the patients, Loss of Interest and Working Capacity in 99% and Anxiety in 96%. (See Table 1). The next three commonest symptoms were, in males, Difficulty in Falling Asleep (Initial Insomnia) 86%, Somatic symptoms of Anxiety 86% and Suicidal symptoms (thoughts and acts) 84%. In females, Fatiguability and Loss of Energy occurred in 91%, Somatic symptoms of Anxiety in 86% and Gastro-Intestinal symptoms in 86%. The last consists predominanly of Loss of Appetite; Constipation is a relatively uncommon symptom. This may seem surprising because most patients will declare that they are constipated. However, if they are asked if the constipation has appeared with the onset of illness or become worse at that time, they will usually say that this is not so, but that the constipation has always been present. In this they are expressing a popular belief rather than describing a true symptom.
If we include the seventh symptom in order of incidence, which is Fatiguability (General Somatic) in males and Suicide in females, we find that symptoms are the same in males and females except that difficulty in falling asleep (Initial Insomnia) in males replaces Loss of Appetite in females. The least common symptoms are the same for both sexes: Hypochondriasis (36% in males and 30% in females) and Loss of Insight (males 30% and females 21%).
Retardation comes fourth in males (62%) and fifteenth in females (44%). Agitation comes fifteenth in males (61%) and eleventh in females (72%). Thus Agitation is as common is males as Retardation but nearly twice as common in females.
One way of comparing the difference in incidence of symptoms between the sexes is by means of the chi-square test. The difference is statistically significant in only three symptoms: Fatiguability (M.81%, F.91%), Retardation (M.62%, F.44%) and Loss of Libido (M. 68%, F. 50%). The last finding is of doubtful significance. The presence of this symptom can be assessed only if there is evidence of deterioration of libido in relation to the illness. Although libido can persist into old age, there is a steady decline and loss with increasing years , so that it becomes progressively more difficult to elicit as a *symptom* in older pa-

Table 1 Frequency of Symptoms

Males		Females	
Item No.	%	Item No.	%
1 Depression	100.0	1 Depression	100.0
7 Loss of Interest	98.9	7 Loss of Interest	99.1
10 Anxiety Psychic	95.7	10 Anxiety Psychic	96.4
4 Insomnia Initial	86.0	13 Somatic General	90.9
11 Anxiety Somatic	86.0	11 Anxiety Somatic	85.5
3 Suicide	83.9	12 Somatic Gas-Intest.	85.5
13 Somatic General	80.6	3 Suicide	83.6
6 Insomnia Delayed	77.4	4 Insomnia Initial	79.1
12 Somatic Gas-Int.	76.3	2 Guilt	78.2
2 Guilt	72.0	6 Insomnia Delayed	76.4
17 Weight Loss	69.9	9 Agitation	71.8
5 Insomnia Middle	68.8	17 Weight Loss	69.1
14 Libido	67.7	5 Insomnia Middle	67.3
8 Retardation	62.4	14 Libido	50.0
9 Agitation	61.2	8 Retardation	43.6
15 Hypochondriasis	35.5	15 Hypochondriasis	30.0
16 Loss of Insight	30.1	16 Loss of Insight	20.9

tients. It is particularly difficult in female patients, partly because sexuality in women is less of a drive and more of a response to stimulation, and partly because an ever increasing proportion of older female patients is widowed. It is very difficult to obtain information about libido in a woman of 60 years who has been widowed for 20 years! In consequence, absence of this symptom signifies only too often mere absence of information.

Another way of comparing the symptoms in the two sexes is to compare their order. Spearman's rank correlation is 0.93, which indicates that although there are minor differences between the sexes in the pattern of symptoms, they are recognisably the same. It would therefore appear that these findings are of little or no interest, but I would draw the attention of clinicians to the importance of Fatiguability as an extremely common symptom in women. It may dominate the clinical picture as presented by the patients.

The foregoing has been concerned with the incidence of symptoms, regardless of whether they are trivial or severe. Bearing in mind the difficulties raised by the differring incidence in the two sexes, we can also compare the mean level of symptoms. Females are significantly more Depressed (t=3.63, p=.001) and Agitated (t=2.72, p=.01). They have a higher level of Psychic Anxiety (t=3.63, p=.001), Somatic symptoms of Anxiety (t=2.38, p=.02), Fatiguability (General Somatic) (t=3.30, p=.01), but less Loss of Libido (t=2.05, p=.01). Once again, the last figure must be interpreted with caution. Finally, there is no overall difference in the level of Severity of Illness as measured by the Total Score on the rating scale (t=1.37, not significant).

Symptomatology in Females

It is now generally accepted that a simple measure of the severity of illness can be obtained by summing the scores on all the symptoms. The justification of this is that all the symptoms are positively correlated, i.e. they have a common variance. Adding the scores on the individual symptoms sums the common variance, but the non-common variance tends to cancel out. One way of measuring the contribution

of each symptom to the total score is to examine its correlation with the total. Of course, it must be borne in mind that the total score also includes the contribution of the individual symptom. It is therefore not suprising that the correlation between individual symptoms and total score are all positive (though this is not necessarily so). For three of them, the correlations fall below the 0.05 level of significance: Somatic symptoms of Anxiety, Hypochondriasis and Loss of Libido. It has been argued that if items in a scale do not contribute significantly to the score, they could just as well be deleted, thereby making the scale shorter and simpler. This is appropriate for items which are uncommon such as Hypochondriasis and Loss of Libido. Indeed, for the last symptom, it is tactful for the clinician to refrain from asking questions on such a subject in older female patients since very little information is lost by such consideration for their feelings. In the case of Somatic symptoms of Anxiety, it would be unwise clinically to omit this item. When these symproms are present they can be a great source of disability to the patient and the clinician must show appropriate interest in them.
The relationship between symptoms are of great interest but cannot be considered here in detail. One symptom in its different forms is of particular interest. Difficulty in falling asleep, i.e. insomnia at the initial period of sleep is usually considered to be associated with anxiety, and early morning awakening, i.e. insomnia delayed until the end of the sleep period, is similarly associated with depression, but in this series, both of these correlations are non-significant. Both, however, are significantly correlated with total score, suggesting that these two symptoms are really functions of the severity of illness. Middle insomnia appears, at first sight, to be no more than an artefact arising from the clinical way of looking at insomnia, but I am now convinced that it is a real symptom in its own right. Many patients report that they have no difficulty in falling asleep but wake during the night in a disturbed state, eventually falling asleep again until the morning. Finally, all the types of disturbance of sleep are positively correlated.
Severity of Illness (Total Score) is not related to Age, the presence or absence of a Family History of Depressive Illness, of Psychological Precipitating Stresses, Obsessional or Neurotic traits of personality, and the number of previous attacks. This last does not accord with the view that "reactive" depressions are milder than the "endogenous" depressions.
"Reactive" depressions are often thought to have a pattern of symptoms different from "endogenous" depressions, but none of the correlations between psychological precipitants and other symptoms reached significant levels (though this is based on a mere 25 cases). Much work has been carried out on symptom patters but the results are far from conclusive. The use of psychometric methods has directed attention to the frequency distribution of rating scale scores. If the two types of depressions did not really differ then it would be expected that the frequency distribution would follow a Gaussian ("normal") distribution. A bimodal distribution would contradict this. In the present data, the distribution of total scores follows a normal curve.
Factor analysis has been used to extract components measuring different "dimensions" from the correlation matrix of the scale items. The first component is clearly a measure of severity of illness. The second component distinguishes between the "retarded" pattern of symptoms and the "anxious-agitated" pattern, though this has not always been confirmed. In the present data, both factors show normal distributions and this is so when they have undergone Varimax rotations. These results are quite different from those of the Newcastle school, who have always found sharply bimodal distributions, e.g. Carney et al. (1965). Why there should be such obvious differences between researchers has not yet been resolved. One suggestion I would like to make is that possibly the syndrome which the Newcastle workers differentiate from "endogenous depression" is that found in the patients I have excluded.
There are similarities and differences between these data and those of Baumann (1976), but there are difficulties in making comparisons. Baumann's data were ob-

tained by many raters and thus lacks the uniformity of the present series. Furthermore, in his series of 197 depressive patients he included 32 diagnosed as "schizoaffective" and 19 patients having "other diagnoses".
Much work has been done in the last decade in Europe on the course of the depressions. Angst et al. (1969) found that the length of an attack of depressive illness (phase) follows a log normal distribution. This signifies that the distribution is asymmetrical, but becomes "normal" when the length of illness is replaced by its logarithm. Their data were derived from retrospective examination of case records. The present work can give information only on the length of the illness up to the time the patient came for treatment. It too follows a log normal distribution.
When questioned about the lenght of illness, many patients have great difficulty in deciding how long they have been ill. Careful questioning indicates that in such cases, the acute phase of illness has been preceded by a milder phase which has sometimes lasted for a number of years. In an important paper by Hays (1964) it was pointed out that the prodromal phase could show symptoms either of depression or "anxiety neurosis". My own experiecnce is that in the latter type, the patients can be quite severely disturbed. My data show that this prodromal phase also follows a log normal distribution. It is of particular interest that it is significantly shorter in females than in males.

REFERENCES

Angst, J., P. Grof, H. Hippius, W. Pöldinger, E. Varga, P. Weis and F. Wyss (1969). Verlaufgesetzlichkeiten depressiver Syndrom. In H. Hippius and H. Selbach (ed.) "Das depressive Syndrom". Urban and Schwarzenberg, Munich.
Baumann U. (1976). Methodische Untersuchungen zur Hamilton-Depression-Skala. Arch. Psychiat. Nervenkr. 222, 359-375.
Carney M.W.P., M. Roth, and R.F. Garside (1965). The diagnosis of depressive syndromes. Brit. J. Psychiat. 111, 659-674.
Hamilton M. (1967). Development of a rating scale for primary depressive illness. Brit. J. Soc. Clin. Psychol. 6, 278-296.
Hays P. (1964). Modes of onset of psychotic depression. Brit. Med. J. 2, 779-784.

Depressive Symptoms in a Greek Population Sample: Investigation with the MMPI

A. Kokkevi, A. Adamou, M. Repapi, M. Typaldou and C. Stefanis

Department of Psychiatry, University of Athens, Eginition Hospital, Athens, Greece

ABSTRACT

Depressive symptoms in adults and adolescents have been studied with the MMPI in a greek semi-urban general population sample.
Elevations of the D scale were found in 16% of adults and 18% of adolescents, mean scores in the D scale being lower for adolescents.
Sex comparisons showed that females had higher elevations in the D scale than males. In adults, the frequency of elevated D scale was higher for women (19%) than for men (12%). In adolescents, on the contrary, D scale elevations were more frequent in boys (21%) than in girls (14%), although the mean D scale scores were lower for boys.
Depressive symptoms were found to be more frequently present and more pronounced in women with elevated (pathological) MMPI profiles. In adolescents with elevated profile, no difference in the frequency of depressive symptoms was observed between boys and girls. Mild depressive symptoms were however predominant in the elevated profiles of boys while in girls intense depressive symptoms were observed. The comparison between adults and adolescents showed that mild depressive symptoms were more frequently met in adolescents than adults as part of their general psychopathological profile.

KEYWORDS

Depressive symptoms; general population; differential prevalence; adults - adolescents; MMPI investigation.

INTRODUCTION

Studies on the prevalence of depressive symptoms in general population samples yielded varying results depending on population (rural or urban), sex, age and the socioeconomic level of the subjects.
The Midtown Manhattan Study in New York during the years 1953-54 (Srole and co-workers, 1962; Langner and Michael, 1963), showed that the 23,6% of the urban population presented depressive symptoms.
In the rural population of Nova Scotia in Canada (Leighton and co-workers, 1963), a 7,2% of the population reported depressive symptoms.
Another study conducted in several counties of Central America (Blumenthal and

co-workers, 1975) revealed depressive symptoms in the 32% of women and the 12% of men.
In a near London area (Martin, 1957), 10% of men and 24% of women presented depressive symptoms. A more recent study, in 1974, on a female working-class population in Camberwell (Brown and Harris, 1978), showed, that 17% of women were suffering from depression and 19% were borderline cases of depression.
In another part of England, the Isle of Wight, Rutter and co-workers (1976) found that a 0,5% of the 2303 fourteen years old population suffered from depression and a 1.3% presented an affective disorder with anxiety and depressive components. The 1/5 of adolescents however, presented some symptoms of mild depression.
In Greece, information on the prevalence of depressive symptoms in general population is still lacking. In this paper preliminary findings on this subject are presented. The data on a general population sample aged 15 to 65 were derived from the ongoing Salamis epidemiological study*
Salamis is an island near the port of Pireus. It takes only 10 minutes by boat to reach the island with very good commuting facilities. Most of its labor force is daily employed in various settings in Pireus. Despite the semi-urban consistency of its 25000 population, Salamis can be considered as part of the Athens greater area.

MATERIAL AND METHODS

Assessment Procedures

The research instrument used was the Minnesota Multiphasic Personality Inventory (MMPI) (Hathaway and McKinley 1967). The greek MMPI version (Kokkevi and co-workers,1979) is currently used in the Department of Psychiatry of Athens University since 1972 with a very good face validity.
The MMPI offers the following advantage as compared to other scales assessing depression: it gives a general "overview" of the subject's psychopathology, and can thus be determined whether depression is a single or a major symptom in the subject's psychopathology or whether it merely contributes to the overall symptomatology of some other than depression mental disorder.
The Depression (D) scale is one of the MMPI's ten basic scales. It comprises 60 statements, most of which concern depressive symptoms (neurotic or psychotic). The scale is sensitive to mood swings and this is one reason for its frequent use in the evaluation of treatment.
A high correlation ($r = .51$ to $.72$) has been found between scores in the scale of Depression and clinical assessments or other measures of depression like the Zung, Beck and Hamilton scales of Depression, (Endicott and Jortner, 1966; Zuckerman and co-workers, 1967; Zung and co-workers, 1965; Zung,1967; Morgan,1968; Schnurr and co-workers, 1976).

Subjects

A total number of 254 subjects were tested. The sample consisted of 137 adults between 20 and 66 years of age (57 males with a mean age of 44 and 80 females with a mean age of 36) and 117 adolescents.
Male subjects had an average of 11,6 years of formal education and females had an average of 12,9 years of formal education.

---

* This study was initiated in 1978 on the population of Salamis island and is coordinated by Dr Kritsikis (Department of Cardiology, Athens University). It is a multidisciplinary longitudinal epidemiological study of the island population. Psychological and psychiatric investigations which are an integral part of this study are carried out by the staff of the Department of Psychiatry of Athens University.

Half of the males were middle or upper level employees, 33% were craftsmen or skilled workers and the rest were small businessmen or students.
Most of the women (59%) were housewives, and most of those who were employed were middle or upper level employees, primarily high-school teachers and some were involved in small businesses.
62 of the adolescents were boys and 55 were girls. All were students and were randomly selected (every third student - of those who completed the test - attending the last three years of high-school).

RESULTS

Findings in the D scale have been separately processed for the two age groups (adults and adolescents) and for the two sexes in the study groups. Raw scores of at least one SD from the mean of the respective age/sex group has been considered as the criterion for elevated D scale.
Table 1 shows the percentages of subjects with elevated D scale, according to their age groups and sex, together with the results of statistical analysis.
In the adult group 16% of subjects present the D scale elevated more than 1SD above their group mean. Most of them (9.5%) have the D scale moderately elevated (2SD>D>1SD) while a smaller percentage (6,5%) have higher elevations (D>2SD).
As to sex differences, in the adult groups the percentage of women with an elevated D scale is higher (18.7% of women, 12.3% of men). Women tend also to present higher elevations of the D scales than men: D>2SD for 7.5% of women and 5.3% of men.
In the adolescent group 18% of subjects present the D scale elevated more than 1SD above their group mean. Most of them (14.5%) show the D scale moderately elevated while the rest (3.4%) show more pronounced elevations (D>2SD).
Regarding sex differences in the adolescent group, more boys than girls present the D scale elevated (21% of boys, 14% of girls). However all boys have the D scale moderately elevated (2SD>D>1SD) while in half of the girls with elevated D scale the elevation is higher (D>2SD). This difference is statistically significant (p<.05).
Differences between the two age groups are observed on the degree of elevation of the D scale. A higher percentage of adolescents than adults present the D scale moderately elevated (14.5% of adolescents, 9.5% of adults) while the percentage of subjects with pronounced elevations of the D scale is higher in the adult group (6.5% in adults, 3.4% in adolescents, p<.01).

TABLE 1: Percentage of Subjects in the General Population Sample with the Depression Scale (D) elevated (Sex and Age Group Differences)

	MEN (N=57) %	WOMEN (N=80) %	x^2	P
D>1SD	12.3	18.7	1.03	n.s.
2SD>D>1SD	7.0	11.2	0.69	n.s.
D>2SD	5.3	7.5	0.27	n.s

	BOYS (N=62) %	GIRLS (N=55) %	x^2	P
D>1SD	21	14	0.82	n.s.
2SD>D>1SD	21	7.3	4.4	.05
D>2SD	0	7.3	4.67	.05

	MEN-WOMEN (N=137) %	BOYS-GIRLS (N=117) %	x^2	P
D>1SD	16	18	1.6	n.s.
2SD>D>1SD	9.5	14.5	1.54	n.s.
D>2SD	6.5	3.4	8.37	.01

Table 2 shows the Mean values in the D scale in the total sample and in the subgroups that have the D scale elevated.
In the total adult group the Mean value in the D scale is 22.98 (SD=5.16) for men and 26.5 (SD=5.46) for women. This difference is statistically significant ($p<.01$). In the total adolescent group the Mean value in the D scale is 19.77 (SD=4.99) for boys and 22.53 (SD=5.48) for girls. This difference is statistically significant ($p<.01$).
The Mean values of the D scale in the adolescent subgroup with elevated D scale are 26.92 (SD=1.5) for boys and 32.5 (SD=4.24) for girls. The difference is statistically significant ($p<.005$).
In the adult group the Mean value of the D scale is 25.04 (SD=5.6) and in the group of adolescents 21.09 (SD=5.38). The difference in the Mean values between adults and adolescents is statistically significant ($p<.001$).
In the subgroup of the adults and adolescents with the D scale elevated, the Mean for adults is 34.14 (SD=3.2) and for adolescents 29.05 (SD=3.92). This difference is again statistically significant ($p<.001$).

TABLE 2: Mean Depression Scale (D) Scores in the Total Sample and in the Subgroups with the D Scale Elevated (Sex and Age-Group Differences)

	MEN		WOMEN		t	p
	M	SD	M	SD		
	(N=57)		(N=80)			
Total Sample	22.98	5.16	26.5	5.46	3.84	.01
	(N=7)		(N=15)			
Subgroups with D Elevated	31.71	2.29	35.27	2.96	3.08	.01

	BOYS M	SD	GIRLS M	SD	t	p
Total Sample	(N=61) 19.77	4.99	(N=55) 22.53	5.48	2.83	.01
Subgroups with D Elevated	(N=13) 26.92	1.5	(N=8) 32.5	4.24	3.58	.005

	MEN - WOMEN M	SD	BOYS - GIRLS M	SD	t	p
Total Sample	(N=137) 25.04	5.6	(N=117) 21.09	5.38	5.75	.001
Subgroups with D Elevated	(N=22) 34.14	3.2	(N=21) 29.05	3.92	4.65	.001

Table 3 shows the percentage of subjects by sex and age group who have an elevated psychological profile (indicating psychopathology) in the MMPI, that is one or more of the 10 basic clinical scales elevated more than 2SD from their respective group mean. The deviations of 2SD from the mean is considered in the evaluation of the MMPI scale elevations as the upper normal limit.
In the adult populations 24.1% (22.8% of men and 25% of women) have an elevated profile. In the adolescent population an elevated profile is found in 18.8% (19.4% of boys and 18.2% of girls).

TABLE 3: Percentage of Subjects with Elevated* Profiles (Sex and Age-group Differences)

MEN (N=57)	WOMEN (N=80)	X^2	P
% 22.8	% 25	0.09	n.s.

BOYS (N=62)	GIRLS (N=55)	X^2	P
% 19.4	% 18.2	0.03	n.s.

MEN - WOMEN (N=137)	BOYS - GIRLS (N=117)	X^2	P
% 24.1	% 18.8	1.04	n.s.

* One or more scales elevated more than 2SD from their respective group mean.

Table 4 shows the relative position of the D scale in the profiles with elevated scales.
In the adult sample, 30.7% (4/13) of men and 45% (9/20) of women who have elevated profiles present also the D scale elevated. In the above profiles the D scale is the highest scale in 7.7% (1/13) of men and 30% (6/20) of women.
In the adolescent sample, 66.7% (8/12) of boys and 70% (7/10) of girls with elevated profiles present also the D scale elevated. The D scale is found as the higher in elevation order scale in 40% (4/10) of girls and none of the boys (0/12). This difference between boys and girls is statistically significant ($p<.05$).
A 39.4% (13/33) and a 68.2% (15/22) of adolescents with elevated profile have the D scale elevated. The difference is statistically significant ($p<.05$). Among these subjects 21.2% (7/33) of adults and 18.2% (4/22) of adolescents present the D scale as the higher scale of their elevated profile.

TABLE 4: The Depression Scale (D) Scores in the Group of Subjects with Elevated* Profiles (Percentage of Subjects with D Scale Elevated, Percentage of Subjects with D scale as the highest Profile Scale).

	MEN (N=13) %	WOMEN (N=20) %	x^2	P
D: elevated	30.7	45	0.67	n.s.
D: the highest profile scale	7.7	30	2.35	n.s.

	BOYS (N=12) %	GIRLS (N=10) %	x^2	P
D: elevated	66.7	70	0.03	n.s.
D: the highest profile scale	0	40	5.87	.05

	MEN - WOMEN (N=33) %	BOYS - GIRLS (N=22) %	x^2	P
D: elevated	39.4	68.2	4.38	.05
D: the highest profile scale	21.2	18.2	0.08	n.s.

* One or more scales elevated more than 2SD from their respective group mean.

DISCUSSION

Mean scores in the Depression scale are higher for females as compared to males, both in adults and in adolescents. This also holds for the subgroup of subjects who have the Depression scale elevated (one SD or more, higher than the mean). The same sex differences were also seen in population samples of other countries where the MMPI has been standardized (U.S.A., Dahlstrom and Welsh, 1960; France, Perse, 1966).
In our samples, females admit a greater number of depressive symptoms as compared to males (19% of the female, 12% of the male subjects). The opposite has been observed in the group of adolescents. Symptoms of depression were admitted more frequently by boys rather than girls (21% of the boys compared to 14% of the girls). The intensity of depressive symptoms (D scale elevations) was however smaller in the adolescent boys than it was in the girls. There were no boys with the D scale elevated more than 2 SDs above their mean score, while of those girls with an elevation on the Depression scale half had elevations of more than 2 SDs above their mean.
There is no difference in the frequency of depressive symptoms between adults and adolescents. What differs seems to be the intensity. Adolescents admit to have significantly fewer symptoms of depression than adults.
Regarding the elevated profiles (that is the profiles with a broader psychopathological picture) no differences are observed between the sexes (23% in men, 25% in women ; 19% in boys, 19% in girls). However adults have more elevated (pathological) profiles compared to adolescents (24% of adults, 19% of adolescents).
In the group of adults with "pathological" profiles, Depression scale elevations were more frequent and higher in women than they were in men (more frequent: 45% in women, 31% in men; peak elevation: 66% of women and 25% of men).
It was also found that mild elevations of the Depression scale are predominant in the general psychopathological picture of boys, while in girls intense depressive symptoms were more frequent (D, highest scale in 40% of girls and 0% of boys). The comparison of adult and adolescent groups have shown that mild elevations in the D scale are more often a part of the general psychopathological picture in adolescent groups than adult groups (68% in adolescents, 39% in adults).
As different assessment methods have been used in the investigation of depressive symptomatology on general population in the various studies mentionned in our introduction (interviews, psychiatric evaluation scales), it is not easy to directly compare our results with those obtained from these studies. However it is worth noticing that despite differences in methodology and population studied the results are in many respects strikingly similar. The percentage of the depressive symptoms admitted by subjects in the general population which we investigated, is in between the percentages mentionned for urban (Martin and co-workers, 1957; Srole and co-workers, 1962; Langner and Michael, 1963; Blumenthal, 1975; Brown and Harris, 1978; Craig and Natta, 1979) and rural areas (Leighton and co-workers, 1963).
Depressive symptoms are more often observed in females than in males as in studies from other countries. The percentage of women with depressive symptoms in our greek sample seems to be lower to that of other countries. Brown and Harris (1978) in Camberwell have found 36% of the women admitting depressive symptoms. Their subjects, however, belonged to the working class while in our sample lower middle class women predominated.
In the adolescent population our findings agree to those of Rutter and co-workers (1976) in England. That is, mild depressive symptoms are much more frequently observed than severe depressive symptoms in adolescents.

REFERENCES

Blumenthal,M.D. (1975). Arch.Gen.Psychiat. 32, 971-978.
Brown,G.W., and T.Harris (1978). Social Origins of Depression. A Study of Psychiatric Disorders in Women. Tavistock, London.
Craig,T.J. and P.A.Van Natta (1979). Arch.Gen.Psychiat. 36, 149-154.
Dahlstrom,W.G., and G.S.Welsch (1960). An MMPI Handbook. University of Minnesota Press, Minneapolis.
Endicott,N.A. and S.Jortner (1966). Arch.Gen.Psychiat. 15, 249-255.
Hathaway,S.R. and J.C. McKinley (1967). The MMPI Manual. The Psychological Corporation. New York.
Kokkevi,A. D.Kyriazis and C.Stefanis (1979). MMPI: Greek Version. Athens University Psychiatric Clinic. Athens.
Langner,T.S. and S.T.Michael (1963). Life Stress and Mental Health: The Midtown Manhattan Study. Free Press, New York.
Leighton,D.C., J.S.Harding, D.B.Macklin, A.M.MacMillan, and A.H.Leighton (1963). The Character of Danger: Psychiatric Symptoms in Selected Communities. The Stirling County Study of Psychiatric Disorder and Sociocultural Environment, Vol.3 .Basic Books, New York.
Martin,F.F.,J.H.F.Brotherston and S.P.W.Chave (1957). Brit.J.Prev.Soc.Med., 11, 196-202.
Morgan,W.P. (1968). Selected Physiological and Psychomotor Correlates of Depression in Psychiatric Patients. In Res. Quart. of the Am. Ass. of Hlth. and Phys. Ed., 39, 1037-1043.
Perse,J. (1966). MMPI: Manuel. Les Éditions du Centre de Psychologie Appliquée, Paris.
Rutter,M., P.Graham, D.Chadwick and W.Yule (1976). J.Child Psychol.Psychiat.,17, 35-56.
Schnurr,R., P.C.Hoaken, and F.S.Jarrett (1976). Can.Psych.Ass.J., 21, 473-476.
Srole,L., T.S.Langner, S.T.Michael, M.K.Opler, and T.A.C.Rennie (1962). Mental Health in the Metropolis: The Midtown Manhattan Study. McGraw-Hill Book Co Inc., New York.
Zuckerman,M.,H.Persky,K.M.Eckman and T.R.Hopkins (1967). J.Proj.Techn.Person. Ass. 31, 39-48.
Zung,W.W., C.B.Richards and M.J.Short (1965). Arch.Gen.Psychiat., 13, 508-515.
Zung,W.W. (1967). Arch.Gen.Psychiat., 16, 543-547.

Sex Differences in Depression: Observations on an Outpatient Psychiatric Sample

M. Markidis, J. Mantonakis, V. Kontaxakis and G. Gournas

Department of Psychiatry, University of Athens, Eginition Hospital, Athens, Greece

ABSTRACT

1. The aim of this retrospective study is to investigate the sex related differences in depression. Results support the view that depression is more prevalent among women than men, though the preponderance of neurotic depression in females is decreasing over time.
2. The possible explanation of these findings are discussed.

KEYWORDS

Sex differential; endogenous depression; involutional depression; neurotic depression; female social role; emancipation.

INTRODUCTION

Depression is more common in women than in men, whether its epidemiological study is based on hospitalized patients or concerns the general population (Kendell, 1970; DeFundia et al, 1971; Dohrenwend, 1975). There are a number of explanations concerning the sex-related differences in depressive diagnosis and some of them are focused on the restricting social female role that tends to increase the experience stresses leading to depression (Kaplan, 1972; Gove and Tudor, 1973). The objective of our retrospective study is to demonstrate the sex differential in depression and its alteration over time, possibly related to changes in the sociocultural conditions and in the roles women occupy in the transitory greek society.

METHODS

First referrals of depressive patients to the Psychiatric Outpatient Department Eginition Hospital during 1969 and 1979 were included in this study. This hospital is indicated for this kind of investigation because of reasons already described (Stefanis et al., 1976). On the basis of the diagnosis given as a result of one or more interviews, these patients were classified into 3 groups, i.e. Endogenous depression (unipolar and bipolar depressive psychosis), involutional depression and neurotic depression. A fourth group includes the unclassified cases, in which depression was the predominant feature but specific diagnosis could not be established at the Outpatient Clinic of the Hospital.

460 patients were diagnosed as depressives during 1969 (27.51% of the general outpatient population) and 397 during 1979 (26.52% of this population). The mean age of onset was 41.0±14.7 years in 1969 (44.5 years for the males and 39.3 years for the females) and 40.5±14.9 years in 1979 (42.0 years for the males and 39.0 years for the females).
The chi-square test was mainly used to detect the sex differences in the sample during the two selected years of the study. The self destructive ideas and tendencies in both males and females were also studied.

RESULTS

The relation of the depressive population to the general outpatient population by sex in 1969 and 1979 respectively is presented on Table 1.

TABLE 1 Relation of depressives to the general Outpatient population by sex, in 1969 and 1979.

Sex	1969 Outpatient population N	%	Depressives N	%	1979 Outpatient population N	%	Depressives N	%
Males	869	52.00	154	33.48	900	60.10	158	39.80
Females	803	48.00	306	66.52	597	39.90	239	60.20
Total	1672		460		1497		397	

While males are significantly more prevalent than females in the general outpatient population of the sample ($p<0.0005$), depressive females are significantly more prevalent than depressive males in 1969 as well as in 1979 (Table 2).

TABLE 2. Depression by sex related to other diagnoses in the general Outpatient population of the sample.

	Depressions N	%	Other diagnoses N	%	General Outpatient population	
1969						
Males	154	17.72	715	82.28	869	N=1672
Females	306	38.11	497	61.89	803	$X^2=86.96$ $p<0.0005$

	Depressions N	%	Other diagnoses N	%	General Outpatient population	
1979						
Males	158	17.56	742	82.44	900	N=1497
Females	239	40.03	358	59.97	597	$X^2=93.06$ $p<0.0005$

The distribution of the depressive sample by sex and diagnostic groups is presented on Table 3. No changes of importance were detected with respect to sex differential in the endogenous depression group between the years studied, though a general increase of the patients thus diagnosed in 1979 was found. Changes with respect to sex differential in the Involutional Depression group were also not significant. Nevertheless, the sex related differences were far from the expected ratio 3:1 of female preponderance (Kielholz, 1959). Changes of significance were found with respect to sex differential in the neurotic depression group, where the prevalence of women decreases from 38.26 per cent to 24.69 per cent over the de-

Sex Differences in Depression

cade studied.

TABLE 3 Distribution of the depressive sample by sex and diagnostic groups.

Year	Sex	Endogenous depression N	%	Involutional depression N	%	Neurotic depression N	%	Unclassified cases N	%	Total N	%
1969	Males	36	7.83	42	9.13	62	13.48	14	3.04	154	33.48
	Females	60	13.04	58	12.61	176	38.26	12	2.61	306	66.52
	Total	96	20.87	100	21.74	238	51.74	26	5.65	460	
1979	Males	49	12.34	41	10.33	61	15.37	7	1.76	158	39.80
	Females	85	21.41	49	12.34	98	24.69	7	1.76	239	60.20
	Total	134	33.75	90	22.67	159	40.06	14	3.52	397	

The same finding concerning the prevalence of the neurotic depression by sex in comparison to the prevalence of the other forms of depression is confirmed in Table 4.

TABLE 4 Neurotic depression by sex and by other forms of depression

Females

	Neurotic depression N	%	Other forms of depression N	%	Total	
1969	176	57.51	130	42.49	306	$N=545$
1979	98	41.00	141	59.00	239	$X^2=14.6353$
						$p<0.0005$

Males

	Neurotic depression N	%	Other forms of depression N	%	Total	
1969	62	40.26	92	59.74	154	$N=312$
1979	61	38.61	97	61.39	158	$X^2=0.0891$
						Non stat.sign.

Table 5 shows that there are no significant differences among housewifes and professional women with neurotic depression over a ten-year period, at least in the limited sample we were able to have some information about their occupation.

TABLE 5 Occupation of women with neurotic depression

	Housewifes N	%	Professional women N	%	Total	
1969	84	60.87	54	39.13	138	$N=234$
1979	55	57.29	41	42.71	96	$X^2=0.3005$
						Non stat. sign.

Finally Tables 6 and 7 show the self-destructive ideas and tendencies of the depressive sample, as expressed during the psychiatric interviews. The total depressive population of the two years tested reveals an increased incidence of such ideas and tendencies in 1979. This increase is statistically significant and is found in both males and females.

TABLE 6 Self-destructive ideas and tendencies of the depressive population in 1969 and 1979.

	Yes		No		Total	
	N	%	N	%		N=857
1969	80	17.39	380	82.61	460	X^2=8.2878
1979	101	25.44	296	74.56	397	p<0.005

TABLE 7 Self-destructive ideas and tendencies of depressives by sex in 1969 and 1979.

Females	Yes		No		Total	
	N	%	N	%		N=545
1969	52	17.00	254	83.00	306	X^2=3.9421
1979	57	23.85	182	76.15	239	p<0.05

Males	Yes		No		Total	
	N	%	N	%		N=312
1969	28	18.18	126	81.82	154	X^2=4.1049
1979	44	27.85	114	72.15	158	p<0.05

DISCUSSION

The results of this study support the view that women are more likely than men to receive a diagnosis of depression, whether it is the neurotic depression, or one of its psychotic forms. This is in accordance with the findings of most authors. Silverman (1968), for instance, notes: "There appears to be no exception to the generalization that depression is more common in women than in men, whether it is the feeling of depression, neurotic depression or depressive psychosis". Kendell (1970) also states: "The greater liability of women to depression is one of the few facts that is established beyond question".
Our findings could certainly reflect a greater tendency of women to admit depression (or, a willingness of clinicians to diagnose depression more often in females) whereas in fact both sexes experience the same degree of depression (Blumenthal, 1975). However, Kaplan (1977) found that depressive males were not significantly different from females in willingness to express their depressive symptoms. Accordingly, sex differential in depression is not likely to be accounted for in terms of self-disclosure tendencies. Furthermore both males and females in our study reveal an increased incidence of self-destructive ideas over time. This findings could not easily be explained, if the given prevalence was a function of the greater tendency on the part of females to admit to depression.
How can this preponderance of female depressives be explained? Some writers believe that biological characteristics of females (endocrine-physiologic processes) increase the probability of depression among women relative to men (Silverman, 1968; Hamburg, 1971). Others assume that because of the social roles women occupy and the nature of stresses they experience, they are more likely to develop emotional problems than men (Kaplan, 1977). Were women to be raised outside the traditional female role and were to experience a different type of socialization, sex differential in depression would be a different one.
We note that in our study female rates of neurotic depression are getting lower in 1979 relative to 1969. There seem to be no significant differences among housewifes and professional women with neurotic depression during this ten-year period. However, a 3.6 per cent of women have chosen a"profession", instead of keeping simply with the "household" and with rearing children. As Yorburg states (Yorburg, 1974), "it is in Household that the female appears to be permitted exclusively the traditional social role and she has the fewer alternatives to self-punitive responses in the face of blameworthy circumstances".

It is well known, that the social phenomenon of "emancipation" of greek women has produced a considerable change to a country, with culture based on traditional values, like Greece (Safilios, 1972; Stefanis et al, 1976). As a result, there is an increased probability that greek women, by adopting behavioral patterns that permit deflection of blame from themselves in the face of self-devaluating circumstances, avoid experience of depression and are going to change the sex differential in it.

Kaplan (1977) writes: "It should be recalled that the conclusions put forth here are based upon data collected in 1966 and therefore refer to socialization experiences at a much earlier point in time. Whether or not current socialization patterns will continue to inhibit deflection of blame from self on the part of females is problematic. To the extent that they do not continue to do so, the sex differential in depression may be expected to change dramatically". Our study agrees with this hypothesis, showing that by time there is a decrease in neurotic depression in females. This finding emphasizes the need for further investigation of the female social role in Greece and perhaps it suggests that slow transformations are taking place in the handling of their inner conflicts.

REFERENCES

Blumenthal, M.D. (1975). Arch. Gen. Psychiat. 32, 971-978.
DeFundia, T.A., J.G. Draguns and L. Phillips (1971).Soc. Psychiatry 6, 11-20.
Dohrenwend, B.P. (1975). Special issue of J. Health Soc. Behav. 16, 365-392.
Gove, W., and J. Tudor (1973). Am. J. Soc. 78, 812-935.
Hamburg, D.A. (1971). Int. Soc. Sci. J. 23, 36-47.
Kaplan, H.B. (1972). The sociology of Mental Illness. New Haven, Conn. College and University Press
Kaplan, H.B. (1977).Gender and Depression: A sociological Analysis of a Conditional Relationship. In W.E.Fann, I. Karakan, A.D. Pokorny and R.L. Williams (Eds), Phenomenology and Treatment of Depression. Spectrum publications, New York.
Kendell, R. (1970) Arch. Gen. Psychiat. 22, 308-318.
Kielholz, P. (1959). Docum. Geigy Acta psychosom. (N. Amer.), No 1, 37
Safilios-Rothschild, C. (1972). Sociological Focus, 5, 71-83.
Silverman, C. (1968). The epidemiology of Depression. Baltimore: John Hopkins Press, 70
Stefanis, C., M. Markidis and G. Christodoulou (1976).Brit. J. Psychiat. 128, 269-275.
Yorburg, B. (1974). Sexual Identity, Sex Roles and Social change. New York, Wiley.

Masked Depression and Immigration

M. G. Madianos

Department of Psychiatry, University of Athens, Eginition Hospital, Athens, Greece

ABSTRACT

The psychopathological symptom distribution of a representative sample of 225 adult Greek immigrants living in New York City was compared to the psychopathological symptom formation of other Ethnic group samples.
The quality of the psychopathological symptoms reported by Latin American or Mediterranean origin samples was characterized by the greater prevalence of depression and somatic manifestations underlying depression especially among recent immigrants.

KEYWORDS

Greek immigrants; psychiatric morbidity; field survey; prevalence study; acculturation.

INTRODUCTION

During the last decades a number of community field surveys have focused attention on the measurement of psychiatric morbidity by the use of self report psychopathological symptom scales including items detecting anxiety, depression and psychosomatic symptomatology. These scales are measuring the respondents psychiatric impairment in general and are not diagnostic tools, (Gurin and others 1960, Srole and others 1962, Leighton and others 1963, Manis and others 1964, Langner 1965, Dohrenwend and Dohrenwend 1969, Myers and others 1971, Engelsmann and others 1971, Weissman and Myers 1978). Several of these community studies included in their sample various Ethnic groups with European or Latin American origin and some of them were found to present higher rates of depression and psychosomatic symtomatology (Srole and others 1962, Dohrenwend and Dohrenwend 1969). The sociocultural influences on the expression of depressive symptomatology have also been studied (Eaton and Weil 1955, Yap 1965, Zung 1972).
The present study aims to investigate the origins of a large number of psychophysiological manifestations detected in a sample of Greek immigrants living in New York City, and compare their symptom distribution to results from other community studies including immigrant populations (Matlin 1965, Lasry 1977).

MATERIAL AND METHOD

A representative sample of 225 adult Greek immigrants, 124 males and 101 females living in New York City was selected for a personal interview by a Greek Psychiatrist and statified by the length of stay in four groups with a mean of 4.7 years ± 3.1, ranging from 6 months up to 13 years of stay in U.S.
The purpose of this field survey was to examine the acculturation influence on mental health status of the Greek immigrants (Madianos 1980). Their mental health status was assessed by the use of a 22 items scale developed by T.Langner for the Midtown Manhattan Study (Langner 1963). This scale classifies the mental status of a person into six categories according to the number of self reported psychopathological symptoms. The 18 out of 22 items are clustered into three clusters of questions attempting to measure anxiety, depression and psychosomatic manifestations.
The qualitative comparison of the Greek immigrant psychopathological symptoms distribution was enabled by the wide use of the 22 items scale in prevalence studies including a variety of Ethnic groups, natives and immigrants (Srole and others 1962, Manis and others 1964, Dohrenwend and Dohrenwend 1961, Langner 1965, Engelsmann 1971, Matlin 1965, Lasry 1977).

RESULTS

Table 1 shows the percentage of psychopathological symptoms to each of the 22 items clustered in three clusters in seven studies including Anglosaxons and other European origin descendents, French Canadians, Native Mexicans, PuertoRicans and Greek immigrants. The symptom formation of the total Greek sample (n.225) is rather similar to the one of the Washington Heights study (Dohrenwend and Dohrenwend 1969), although a higher number of Greek immigrants tended to feel "isolated apart" and considered themselves as "worrying types".
The distribution of self reported psychosomatic symptoms are twice as often by native Mexicans, native PuertoRicans, French Canadians, than by Anglosaxons and other European origin descendents (Srole and others 1962, Manis and others 1964, Dohrenwend and Dohrenwend 1969).
The 22 item average score of Greek immigrants is 2.50 compared to 5.99, 4.57 and 4.61 of Mexicans, French Canadians and PuertoRicans respectively.

TABLE 1: Percentage of Psychopathological Symptoms to each of the 22 Items Clustered in Three Clusters in Seven Studies.

	Srole Midtown Manhat. Var.Ethn. groups n=1660	Manis Michigan Nat.Amer. n=1183	Dohrenwend Washington Heights Var.Ethn. groups n=1686	Langner Mexico city Mexicans n=302	Engelsmann Montreal French Canadians n=346	Matlin Puerto Rico Puerto Ricans n=713	Madianos New York Greeks n=225
Depression							
Cannot get going	16.4	49.9	12.1	52.7	39.0	33	12.9
Nothing worth	26.7	29.3	15.6	63.9	25.4	43	12.0
Things turn wrong	11.3	11.2	11.5	32.8	32.7	41	14.7
Isolated apart	18.3	17.9	13.9	12.2	24.9	27	27.1
Low spirits	6.7	0.8	5.1	19.9	2.3	24	3.2

Recent Greek immigrants with up to 6 years of stay in U.S.A. tend to over report psychosomatic manifestations and express depressive symptomatology compared to old and second generation immigrants. On the other hand Jewish immigrants express more psychopathological symptoms of anxiety and depression than any of the Greek and PuertoRican respondents.
The Greek immigrant survey questionnaire also included 13 additional items on psychopathology issues. A supplementary analysis of these items showed that: 1) 20% of the total sample reported having sleep disturbances, 2) 34 persons (19%) reported that "their life was useless and nothing was interesting." 24 out of those 34 reported four and over psychopathological symptoms in the Langner Scale, 3) 8 persons were feared that something serious event (death, illness) could hapened to them, 4) 5 females and 3 males expressed a suicidal tendency reporting 8 and over psychopathological symptoms in the Langner scale, four of them had a history of previous suicide attempt during their stay in U.S. The extensive psychiatric interview identified 8 cases, 2 males and 6 females, diagnosed as suffering from depressive illness, with an average of 8.62 (± 3.37) psychopathological symptoms in the Langner scale. All of them were recent immigrants in New York City.

DISCUSSION

The quality of the psychopathological symptoms reported by Latin American or Mediterranean origin populations including immigrants and revealed by the use of the 22 items scale is characterized by the greater prevalence of depression and psychosomatic complaints especially among recent immigrants. This in fact coincides with similar findings reported by other investigations (Langner 1965, Alodi 1971, Haberman 1976).
The question of the somatization phenomena in immigrant and other Ethnic groups has been answered by several authors. Tyhurst (1951) stated that the complaints tend to be expressed in terms of somatic symptoms rather than subjective feelings reflecting modes of expressions culturally influenced.
Others consider somatization of anxiety as the posssible pathogenetic mechanism of the somatic symptoms (Lasry 1973).
This somatization theory is based upon the psychodynamic view of somatization of intrapsychic conflicts as an immature defence mechanism related not only with the patients inability to communicate with the therapist, but also with a somatic orientation toward psychiatric symptoms. Hollingshead and Redlich (1958), tried to give a similar explanation when they observed higher rates of somatic manifestations among lower social class population in their study.
In contrary, others state that somatization is a part of a syndrome called "vital depressive" disorders syndrome with various somatic manifestations in different parts of the body, considered as part of the nuclear depression (Weitbrecht 1963, Kuhn 1972). Angst (1973) postulates that masked depression belongs to the culture independent core of depressive symptomatology as identified from cross-cultural studies and therefore the term "somatization and somatic anxiety" presupposes that physical manifestations are secondarily expressed by preexisting state of anxiety whereas those symptoms are probably primary.
In conclusion it seems that the main characteristic of immigrants psychopathology is anxiety, depression and its somatic equivalents.
A possible pathogenetic mechanism of depression experienced during immigration implicates acculturation stress through a process of acculturation efforts by the immigrant in order to obtain an unsuccessful social acceptance by the natives, feeling of frustration, increased toward the others causing frustration. In many cases this aggression is self directed, causing depression, (Dollard and others 1939, Madianos 1980).

Anxiety
Worrying type	47.1	43.4	37.7	63.9	53.2	60	36.8
Restlessness	18.6	29.7	14.9	37.1	54.3	36	18.6
Personal Worries	20.2	15.9	13.1	29.1	23.7	29	15.1
Nervousness	18.1	23.3	11.4	19.2	25.4	16	20.0
Hands shaking	1.8	3.0	1.6	7.3	3.5	6	1.8

Psychosomatic
Feel weak all over	9.1	9.2	8.7	17.5	26.0	24	11.5
Hot all over	16.3	16.5	14.9	34.8	35.3	38	10.7
Acid stomach	10.1	14.9	9.8	31.1	15.6	39	11.1
Headaches	10.9	11.1	6.8	14.9	11.9	18	8.0
Breathing diffic.	4.0	4.9	3.4	4.6	12.4	6	3.6
Heart beating	3.7	5.8	3.0	5.6	10.1	6	3.6
Cold sweats	2.2	1.9	2.2	15.9	2.0	5	0.9
Fainting spells	1.5	3.4	1.8	4.0	2.0	15	0.4

Ambiguous items
Fullness in head	14.3	17.3	11.4	30.5	18.8	30	4.9
Trouble getting to sleep	14.9	10.2	11.5	8.9	21.1	13	9.3
Memory not all right	6.1	9.5	4.8	21.5	12.1	10	1.8
Poor appetite	4.7	3.1	3.9	4.0	4.9	14	4.5
22 items average score	2.83	3.25	2.18	5.39	4.57	4.61	2.50

Another comparison of the item to item symptom distribution between the Greek sample broken down in four subsamples according to their length of stay in U.S.A. and North African Jewish immigrants in Montreal and PuertoRican immigrants in New York (Washington Heights) is shown in table 2).

TABLE 2: Percentage Distribution of Respondents Reporting Psychopathological Responses to each of the 22 Items in Greek (four groups), Jewish and Puerto Rican Immigrants.

	Greeks (New York City) n 225				Jewish (Montreal) n 480	Puerto Ricans (Wash.Heights N.Y.C.) n 169
	Very Rec. n=51	Recent n=56	Old n=55	Sec.Gen. n=53		
Depression cluster						
Cannot get going	15.6	16.	9.2	11.3	33.2	18
Nothing worth	7.8	16.	10.8	13.2	31.0	27
Things turn wrong	21.5	18	10.8	9.4	22.3	14
Isolated apart	35.2	30.4	23.1	20.7	19.4	20
Low spirits	1.9	1.8	-	9.4	5.4	10
Anxiety cluster						
Worrying type	35.3	39.2	32.3	41.5	64.2	51
Restlessness	19.6	17.9	26.1	9.4	49.6	15
Personal worries	21.5	16.	13.9	9.4	39.2	20
Nervousness	21.5	27.8	18.5	13.2	35.2	14
Hands shaking	1.9	3.5	1.5	-	2.5	-
Psychosomatic cluster						
Feel weak allover	15.6	14.2	12.3	3.8	35.9	14
Hot all over	19.6	16.0	4.6	3.8	30.1	30
Acid stomach	13.7	16.0	7.7	3.8	18.2	15
Headaches	7.8	3.5	1.5	7.5	18.1	7
Breathing diffic.	9.8	10.7	6.2	1.9	11.9	11
Heart beating	7.8	3.6	3.1	-	10.0	2
Cold sweats	-	1.8	1.5	-	2.1	2
Fainting spells	1.9	-	-	-	1.3	3
Ambiguous items						
Fullness in head	9.9	7.2	1.5	1.9	30.0	17
Trouble getting to sleep	9.8	7.2	13.8	5.7	18.0	11
Memory not all right	-	1.8	1.5	1.9	11.5	7
Poor appetite	13.7	1.8	1.5	-	4.8	5
22 items average score	3.05	2.89	3.32	1.81	4.93	2.9

In our sample, the group of very recent Greek immigrants, with a range of 6 to 24 months of stay in U.S.A. showed greater mental health impairment, exactly because the phase of the first "happy days" is succeeded by the phase of ego crises and nostalgia or acculturation stress, frustration and depression.
This view is supported by other immigrant studies, conducted in W.Germany (Haring Xenakis 1973, Cranach 1976). The wide range of physical complaints exhibited by the recent Greek immigrants being in the lower socio-economic class maybe is explained by the somatization of their intrapsychic conflicts and their inability to express them in a different way, if we accept the psychodynamic aspect of masked depression, or by the pathogenetic mechanisms of nuclear depression. The risk for a recent immigrant's exposure into stressors is higher and the probability of exhibiting an affective illness in a form of masked depression is greater resulting in diagnostic problems frequently.

REFERENCES

Alodi,F. (1971). The Italians in Toronto: Mental Health problems of an immigrant community in W.E.Mann (Ed.) Social Deviance in Canada. Toronto.
Angst,J. (1973). Masked depression viewed from cross-cultural standpoint in P.Kielholz (Ed.) Masked Depression. Huber,Bern.
Cranach,M. (1976). Psychiatric disorders among foreign workers in Federal Republic of Germany. Fragen den transkulturell - vergleichenden Psychiatrie in Europa, Kiel.
Dohrenwend,B.P. and B.S.Dohrenwend (1969). Social Status and Psychological Disorder: A causal inquiry. J.Wiley, New York.
Dollard,J., N.Miller, L.Doeb, O.Mowrer,and R.Sears (1939). Frustration and Agression, Yale Univ.Press, New Haven.
Eaton,J.W. and R.J.Weil (1955). Culture and Mental Disorders. Free Press, Clenroe, Ill.
Engelsmann,F.,H.B.M.Murphy, R.Prince, M.Leduc,and H.Demers (1972). Soc. Psychiat. 7, 150-156.
Gurin,G.,J.Veroff,and J.Felds (1960). Americans View Their Mental Health. Basic Books, New York.
Haberman,P. (1976). Ethnicity 3, 133-144.
Haring,C.,C.Xenakis (1973). Nostalgische Reaktionen bei griechischen Gastarbeiten in West Berlin. Fragen den transkulturell-vergleichenden Psychiatrie in Europa, Kiel.
Hollingshead,A.B. and F.C.Redlich (1958). Social Class and Mental Illness. J.Wiley, New York.
Kuhn,R. (1972). Discussion in P.Kielholz (Ed.) Depressive Illness. Huber,Bern.
Langner,T. (1962). J.Hlth.Hum.Beh. 3, 269-276.
Langner,T.S. (1965). Psychophysiological symptoms and the status of women in two Mexican communities in J.Murphy and A.H.Leighton (Ed.) Approaches to Cross-Cultural Psychiatry. Cornell Univ.Press, Ithaca,N.Y.
Lasry,J.C. (1977). Soc.Psychiatry 12, 49-55.
Leighton,D.C.,J.S.Harding, D.B.Macklin, A.M. MacMillan,and A.H.Leighton (1963). The character of danger. Vol.3, BasicBooks, New York.
Madianos,M. (1980). Acculturation and Mental Health of Greek immigrants in U.S.A. Doctoral Dissertation, Athens University Medical School, Athens.
Manis,J.G.,M.J.Brawer,C.L.Hunt,and L.C.Kercher (1964). Am.Soc.Rev. 29, 84-89.
Matlin,N. (1965). The Demography of Happiness. Series 3, San Juan University of PuertoRico Department of Public Health. PuertoRico Master Sample Survey of Health and Welfare.

Myers,J., J.Lindenthal, and M.Pepper (1971). J.Nerv.Ment.Dis. 152, 149-157.
Tyhurst,L. (1951). Am.J.Psychiat. 101, 561-568.
Weissman,M. and J.Myers (1978). Acta Psychiat.Scand. 57, 219-231.
Weitbrecht,H.J. (1963). Psychiatrie in Grundrib. Springer, Berlin.
Yap,P. (1965) Phenomenology of affective disorder in Chinese and other cultures in A.V.Renck R.Porter (Ed.) Transcultural Psychiatry. Churchill, London.
Zung,W.W. (1972). J.Cult.Psychol. 3, 117-183.

4. Biological Aspects of Depression

Recent Advances in the Biology of Depression

W. E. Bunney, Jr. and B. L. Garland

Biological Psychiatry Branch, National Institute of Mental Health, Bethesda, Maryland 20205, USA

ABSTRACT

1. Many new advances have been made in the biology of depression in the past five years. The role of carbamazepine may become more important as a new treatment strategy, especially since some patients who respond to carbamazepine are non-responsive to lithium. The prophylactic properties of carbamazepine have been described in a subgroup of treatment resistant rapid cyclers.
2. The antidepressant effects of sleep deprivation have been reviewed, although the mechanism of action is still unclear. Several groups have shown good antidepressant responses to partial sleep deprivation. However, the effects are transient, lasting only 24-48 hours.
3. The role of endorphins in mental illness is not very well defined, although pain studies indicate that some subgroups of depressed patients may have differential pain sensitivities as compared to normals. Recent techniques for measuring CSF opiate activity may shed some light on the role of opiates in manic vs. depressive episodes. Preliminary evidence indicates a higher level of opiate activity during mania.
4. Low dose dopamine agonists have been used to successfully treat some manic patients. Low doses of drugs such as apomorphine and piribedil have been postulated to affect the presynaptic receptor.
5. The measurement of neuroendocrine levels has consistently demonstrated an abnormal "escape response" to overnight dexamethasone suppression in approximately 40-50% of patients with endogenous depression.
6. The hypothesis that there may be a supersensitive dopamine receptor system in the initial phases of mania, and the finding that lithium can block the development of supersensitive receptors in animals, suggests a possible mechanism for its efficacy in manic-depressive illness.

KEYWORDS

Carbamazepine; sleep deprivation; endorphins; low dose dopamine antagonists; neuroendocrine levels; supersensitive dopamine receptor system.

INTRODUCTION

The advent of new potential treatment strategies in depression has raised exciting possibilities for future research. Current novel therapeutic approaches will be reviewed including the use of carbamazepine, an anticonvulsant medication as an alternative to lithium treatment, the use of forms of sleep deprivation in depression, the administration of opiate compounds and the use of low dose dopamine agonists. This chapter will review recent psychobiological studies in affective illness as they relate to new areas of research.

Carbamazepine

In the mid-1960's much attention was drawn to the anticonvulsant, carbamazepine (Tegretol) when epileptic patients described themselves as feeling brighter and more alert and showed improvement in the affective symptoms of anxiety, irritability, and depression (Dalby, 1975). In open clinical studies, investigators reported that carbamazepine was effective in 55% of 64 manic patients and in 3 of 9 depressed patients (Okuma et al., 1975). In the first placebo-controlled, double-blind experiment, Ballenger and Post (1978) reported improvement in 7 of 9 manic patients and in 5 of 13 depressed patients treated with carbamazepine. One patient, a 39-year-old woman with a 10-year history of manic-depressive illness, and a poor responder to lithium, was administered carbamazepine for a manic episode and showed improvement within two days. When placebo was substituted, she became hypomanic within 36 hours and had a full-blown mania within 72 hours. Upon re-administration of carbamazepine, she improved markedly after three days and remained well while on the medication. However, not all of the carbamazepine responders became worse on placebo; two of the seven manics did not relapse and 2 out of 3 depressed patients showed no relapse. In another study, Okuma et al., 1979, conducted a double-blind trial in which either carbamazepine or chlorpromazine was administered to a total of 60 patients. Of the 32 manic patients receiving carbamazepine, 70% showed improvement in their manic symptomatology. Three groups of investigators have noted a prophylactic effect of carbamazepine in recurrent manic-depressive patients, some of whom had been poor responders to lithium (Okuma et al., 1973, 1979; Takazaki and Hanakoa, 1971; Ballenger and Post, 1978, 1980). Okuma et al. (1973) reported 71% prophylaxis of recurrent mania and 64% prophylaxis of recurrent depression in a sample of 33 patients. Ballenger and Post (1980) reported evidence of prophylaxis in two depressed patients and two manic patients. Preliminary evidence from Okuma et al. (1975,1979) seems to suggest that concomitant treatment with either neuroleptics or lithium may enhance the prophylactic properties of carbamazepine. A low incidence of side effects to carbamazepine treatment has been reported (Okuma et al., 1979 and Ballenger and Post, 1980) when compared to lithium or neuroleptics, thus suggesting that it may be a relatively "nontoxic" substance.

Sleep Deprivation

One of the primary symptoms of depression is a disturbance in sleep. Numerous EEG studies of the sleep-wake cycle indicate that in depressed patients REM sleep occurs earlier in the sleep period than it does in controls (Kupfer et al., 1976; Vogel et al., 1980). The antidepressant effects of sleep deprivation in depression have been reviewed (Gerner et al., 1979); however, the mechanism of action of one night's total sleep loss remains unclear. In medication-free patients the response appears to be short-acting, usually lasting for a period of 24-48 hours (Matussek et al., 1974; van der Burg and van den Hoofdakker, 1975; Post et al., 1976; Schmocker et al., 1975). In contrast, patients treated concomitantly with psychoactive drugs, or in the withdrawal phases of medication, have been reported to have prolonged antidepressant responses following sleep deprivation (Pflug, 1976; Voss and kind, 1974; Loosen et al., 1976; van Scheyen, 1977).

Several investigators have used various types of sleep loss in an effort to behaviorally define the mechanism of the antidepressant effect. Shilgen and Tolle (1980) awakened 30 endogenously depressed patients in the second half of the evening (after approximately four hours of sleep) and kept them awake until the following evening. They reported a 75% improvement in depression. Another group of investigators measured the amount of improvement following partial sleep deprivation to predict responses to lofepramine, a tricyclic compound (Phillip and Werner, 1979). Several studies have used REM deprivation as a means of alleviating depression by arousing subjects at the onset of REM (Vogel, 1975; Vogel et al., 1980). It is possible that the REM suppressant action of monoamine oxidase inhibitors (Wyatt et al., 1977) may relate to their therapeutic mode of action. Tricyclic compounds (Toyoda, 1964; Ritvo, 1967; Hartmann, 1968) have also been associated with REM suppression. Disturbances in circadian rhythms have been suggested as possible causes of sleep abnormalities. Wehr et al. (1979) observed four depressed patients and noted that their time of awakening advanced as they emerged from depression. These investigators subsequently advanced the sleep period of patients and reported an improvement in three out of four. One subject, a 57-year-old depressed woman was brought out of depression twice for a two-week period by advancing her sleep period so that she went to sleep and arose 6 hours earlier than usual. However, subsequent phase advances were not successful in terminating her depression.

Garland and Bunney (unpublished data) compared two types of total sleep loss in drug-free depressed patients by reviewing those patients who were sleep deprived (enforced total sleep loss) and compared them to patients who spontaneously remained awake for a 24-hour period. There was a signigicant improvement in depressive symptoms following sleep deprivation (15 our of 22 patients or 68.2%) as compared with spontaneous sleep loss (4 out of 20 or 20% showed improvement). In agreement with other investigations, however, the antidepressant effects did not last more than 24-48 hours in either group.

Endorphins in Mental Illness

There have been conflicting reports concerning the efficacy of both endorphins and naloxone and their respective roles in mania and depression. Fink et al., (1970) was first to report an antidepressant response to cyclazocine, a mixed opiate agonist-antagonist. In an open clinical trial of chronic severely depressed patients, Fink et al., (1970) reported improvement in 8 our of 10 patients receiving cyclazocine (1.0-3.0 mg/day) within a 4-week period. However, other investigators using either opiate agonists or antagonists were unable to confirm this finding. Terenius et al., (1977) administered naloxone (0.4-0.8 mg t.i.d.), an opiate antagonist, to five depressed patients for a duration of 6-12 days. They observed no positive effects on mood but did note an abrupt worsening of symptoms in two cases following the discontinuation of treatment. Furthermore, they reported that Fraction I endorphin levels were decreased in every session following naloxone treatment; in two cases the decrease was greater that 50%. In another study, Davis et al., (1977) did not see improvement in mood in four depressed patients following acute administration of naloxone.

The effects of beta-endorphin, an opiate agonist, in depression have been equally inconclusive. Angst et al. (1979) administered beta-endorphin (10 mg i.v.) to four bipolar and two unipolar severely depressed hospitalized patients in a non-blind drug trial. In three of the six patients a switch into hypomania or mania was observed during or after the trial. In another study, Kline et al., (1977) and Kline and Lehmann (1979) administered 1.8 - 9.0 mg beta-endorphin to one unipolar and one bipolar depressed patient and noted a transient improvement in both patients. Recently Gerner et al. (1980) reported significant double-blind improvement to beta-endorphin (1.4-10 mg: .02 -.20 mg/kg) in ten depressed patients. Pickar et al. (in press), also using double-blind methodology, however, found no significant effect of beta-endorphin (4-10 mg: .06-.22 mg/kg) in four depressed patients. Neit-

her group observed the occurence of mania or hypomania associated with beta-endorphin administration.
Several groups of investigators hypothesized a greater role for opiated in mania as compared to depression, mainly because opiates have been noted to induce behaviors in normals which are similar to those observed in mania: hyperactivity, increased arousal, grandiosity and euphoria. In a double-blind, placelo-controlled experiment, Janowsky et al., (1979) administered naloxone (20 mg) to 7 manic patients. Two of the patients were on lithium alone while two others received antipsychotic medication in addition to lithium. Results indicated that although there appeared to be an antimanic response to naloxone, only two manic patients showed dramatic changes. However, Emrich et al., (1979) were unable to demonstrate any naloxone-induced changes in two manic patients with doses of 4 and 24.8 mg, respectively. Davis et al. (in press) showed that there were no significant effects of naloxone in 10 manic patients.
The measurement of CSF fractions of endogenous opiates has opened up many new doors for future research, although without the specific identification of the fractions, very little can be concluded as to what role, if any, each may play in affective illness. Lindstrom et al., (1978) reported greater opioid activity during the manic phase as compared to the depressive phase in medicated patients. Pickar et al., (1980) collected samples over a 3-month period from a rapidly cycling manic-depressive (BP II) 57-year-old woman with a 25-year history of affective illness who had been off medication for a period of 21 days. There was a significantly higher level of opioid activity during the manic as compared to the depressed phase.
Behavioral measures of pain perception show that there is greater analgesia in depression as compared to controls (Hemphill et al., 1952; Hall and Stride, 1954; Von Knorring, 1975; Merskey, 1965), with one study showing that analgesia to shock stimuli was more than two standard deviations below normals in a subgroup of the patients (Davis et al., in press). Depressed patients have also been noted to have a high frequency of somatic complaints. In a preliminary study, Davis et al., (in press) correlated the rate of somatic complaints with pain sensitivity and found that depressed patients who rated themselves as having "high distress scores" were more pain insensitive on a psychophysical task than patients with low scores.

Low Dose Dopamine Agonists

Another approach to the treatment pf mania is the administration of low dose dopamine agonists, such as apomorphine and piribedil, which have been shown in animal studies to produce sedation (Strombom, 1976) by possibly inhibiting dopamine-mediated transmission at the presynaptic receptor (Carlsson, 1975). Preliminary data in two of three manic patients suggests that low dose piribedil (20-60 mg/day) is associated with behavioral inhibition and antimanic effects, while higher doses (180-240 mg/day), which are postulated to affect the postsynaptic receptor, were associated with antidepressant effects (Post et al., 1976, 1978) and the activation of recurrent manic episodes in one patient (Post et al., 1978).
Apomorphine in low doses (1 mg) was administered intramuscularly by Corsini et al., (1977) to seven manic patients and was associated with improvement in 3 of 7 patients. However, the effect was temporary, lasting only 20-50 minutes, after which the patients returned to their previous psychotic conditions.

Neuroendocrines

The measurement of neuroendocrine levels in manic-depressive illness has provided some clues to the underlying pathology in some individuals, one of which may involve the hypothalamic-pituitary-adrenal (HPA) cortical axis. In approximately 40-50% of patients with endogenous depression, investigators have documented an abnormal "escape" response to overnight dexamethasone suppression tests, i.e., there is decreased suppression of plasma cortisol levels in response to an overnight

dose of synthetic glucocorticoid dexamethasone, whereas in other psychiatric disorders, less than 5% of the patients showed the abnormal lack of suppression (Carroll, 1978). In further studies attempts were made to clinically characterize the abnormal responders, however the results do not support any particular clinical profile (Carroll and Davies, 1970; Brown et al., 1979 and Schlesser et al., 1969) other than the distinction between endogenous vs. non-endogenous depression (Carroll et al., 1980). Further studies have described genetic contributions in unipolar depressions with the highest frequencies (82%) of abnormal responders occuring in those with familial pure depressive disease (Schlesser et al., 1979). However, Carroll et al. (1980) could not replicate this study in 14 patients using techniques similar to Schlesser et al. (1979).
In another study, Brown et al., (1979) attempted to use the response to the dexamethasone tests as a predictor of treatment outcome. In a sample of 19 patients with primary major depressive disorder, eight (42%) were found to be abnormal responders. Of the eight "escapers", four were treated with desimipramine or imipramine and were reported to show considerable improvement. The remaining four "escapers" treated with amitriptyline and clomipramine showed little or no improvement. The reverse was true in the "suppressor" group, where the significant improvement occured with amitriptyline or chlorimipramine. The authors suggest that depressed patients who do not show pituitary adrenal suppression with dexamethasone might be noradrenaline deficient and that depressed patients who show suppression may be serotonin deficient.
Several other groups of investigators have analyzed other endocrine changes in depression compatible with the dexamethasone suppression data. These include increased cortisol production rates (Gibbons, 1964; Sachar et al., 1970), elevated urinary-free cortisol secretion (Sachar et al., 1973) and increased urinary 17-hydroxycorticosteroid levels (a major breakdown product of cortisol) (Bunney et al., 1965b).
It has been suggested that growth hormone secretion is stimulated by NE agonists and inhibited by NE antagonists through the growth hormone releasing factor (Brown and Reichlin, 1972; Martin 1970), although there is some dopaminergic involvement (Muller et al., 1970; Woolf et al., 1979). In depressed patients, growth hormone responses have been reported to be decreased in response to stimulatory tests, including insulin-bound hypoglycemia (Gregoire et al., 1977; Gruen et al., 1975), L-DOPA (Sachar et al., 1972; Gold et al., 1975) and d-ampheramine (Langer et al., 1976). However, the decrease in GH levels have also been reported in mania (Gold et al., 1975; Casper et al., 1977; Rotrosen, 1978).
Other neuroendocrine levels which have been measured include prolactin and TSH in response to thyrotropin-releasing hormone (TRH) administration. However, these results have been inconsistent (Mendlewicz, 1980; Maeda et al., 1975, 1979; Linnoila et al., 1979; Ehrensing, 1974). Additional studies which measure the release of thyrotropin (TSH) in respone to TRH have also been incoclusive (Prange et al., 1972; Gold et al., 1977; Kirkegaard et al., 1978; Maeda et al., 1975).
The relatively few endocrinological studies in mania suggest that there is normal (Schwartz et al., 1966) or reduced (Rizzo et al., 1954; Bryson and Martin, 1954; Bunney et al., 1965a) adrenal cortical activity. Growth hormone levels in response to insulin or dopamine agonist challenges have been reported by three groups of investigators (Gold et al., 1975; Casper et al., 1977; Rotrosen, 1978) to be decreased in mania.

The Possible Role of Dopamine in the Switch Process

One of the most striking behavioral phenomena in manic-depressive illness is the switch from a retarded depression into a hyperactive manic condition. This can occur during a period of days to minutes (Bunney et al., 1972). We have hypothesized that the switch may be associated with the release of a neurotransmitter that is amplified by a supersensitive neuronal receptor (Bunney et al., 1977a). Lithium might act in the manic-depressive process by blocking the development of supersensitive neuronal receptors. The following data are supportive of such an hypothesis.

Clinical data. The behavior observed during the onset of mania is compatible with a sudden marked functional increase in a released neurotransmitter. This behavior is similar to and at times indistinguishable from behavior associated with the i. v. infusion of a large dose of amphetamine. Bipolar patients often switch from a retarded nonverbal dozing depression into hyperactive mania. This is associated with a sudden marked increase in motor and verbal activity, intrusiveness, increased interest in sex and absense of sleep. Similarly, behavioral changes associated with relatively high doses of i.v. amphetamine include increased motor and verbal activity, increased interest in sex and decreased sleep. Amphetamine increases release and decreases reuptake of catecholamines, particularly dopamine and norepinephrine, thus producting indirect catecholamine agonist actions. While amphetamine rarely produces typical mania, it does provide a drug model that produces both functional increases in brain catecholamines and many behavioral symptoms seen at the onset of mania. It is not suggested that i.v. amphetamine is a model of mania, but only that i.v. amphetamine, which increases brain catecholamine, produces behavioral characteristics that are similar in action to the onset of mania (Bunney et al., 1977b).
Measurements of catechol- and indoleamines and their metabolites have been completed in the urine and CSF over the past decade, during both manic and depressive phases of the illness. In reviewing this data, it is difficult to explain the sudden onset of mania on the basis of a marked release of indole- or catecholamines as reflected by the metabolites, MHPG in the urine and the CSF, and HVA and 5-HIAA in the CSF (Bunney et al., 1977a). The most that can be said is that some authors have reported a moderate increase in these amines in patients who switch from depression into mania. However, the levels in mania do not appear to exceed those noted in normal controls. Recent investigations demonstrated low urinary MHPG levels to be associated with tricyclic-induced switches from depression into mania (Zis et al., 1979). The authors hypothesize that the low MHPG levels, compatible with decreased central norepinephrine turnover, may reflect increased postsynaptic noradrenergic receptor sensitivity. Thus, if one is to hypothesize that mania is associated with a marked increase in functional catecholamine activity, additional mechanisms, such as receptor sensitivity changes, should be considered in a primary or adjunctive role.
Although pharmacological data accumulated in the past suggests a role for NE in mania (Post et al., 1978), recent data has also documented a role for dopamine in the manic process. Briefly, administration of the catecholamine precursor L-DOPA has been reported to be associated with hypomania in bipolar patients (Murphy et al., 1971). However, fusaric acid, which is a dopamine-beta-hydroxylase inhibitor, was not effective in decreasing manic symptomatology (Sack and Goodwin, 1974), thus suggesting that dopamine rather than NE may be involved in mania, since blockade prior to the formation of DA and NE is effective; blocking synthesis following the formation of dopamine and prior to the formation of NE is ineffective in decreasing mania. Finally, pimozide, the most specific neuroleptic blocker of dopamine receptors, has been shown to be effective in decreasing manic symptomatology (Post et al., (1980)).

Animal studies showing blocking of the development of neuronal supersensitivity with lithium carbonate. We would predict that if the development of supersensitive neuronal receptors is important at the point of onset of mania, then the drug that is most effective in preventing the onset of manic episodes, lithium carbonate, might prevent the development of supersensitivity. Thus, the following studies in rats were undertaken.
These studies were stimulated by both our own clinical work and the observations of Klawans (1976), who reported that lithium blocked increased stereotypy induced by apomorphine in rats after treatment with chlorpromazine. Chronic treatment

Recent Advances in the Biology of Depression

with neuroleptics, tyrosine hydroxylase inhibitors, reserpine, or interruption of dopaminergic transmission by lesions of the nigrostriatal dopamine pathway, have been shown to produce an increased sensitivity to the behavioral effects of drugs that stimulate dopamine receptors. Supersensitivity induced by chronic administration of neuroleptics (Muller and Seeman, 1978; Burt et al., (1977) as well as nigrostriatal lesions (Creese et al., 1977) have recently been found to be accompanied by an increase in striatal dopamine receptor sites. It has been proposed that this apparent proliferation of receptors following chronic blockade of dopaminergic transmission may be causally related to behavioral supersensitivity (Burt et al., 1977; Creese et al., 1977).
In our own work (Pert et al., 1978), long-term treatment of rats with haloperidol produced a statistically significant increased sensitivity to the locomotor and stereotypic effects of the dopamine agonist apomorphine. Haloperidol administration was also accompanied by increased ^{3}H-spiroperidol binding in the striatum. However, the rats treated with lithium one week before and during haloperidol administration failed to develop the behavioral sensitivity response to apomorphine (as measured by locomotor and stereotypic effects), and the increased striatal dopamine receptor binding. Scatchard analysis of this data revealed that the increase in receptor binding of the haloperidol-treated group was due to an increase in the number of binding sites and not an alteration in the affinities of the existing binding sites. It was also shown that lithium did not increase the rate of haloperidol excretion or decrease the concentration of haloperidol at the dopamine receptors in the rat striatum.
In addition to the behavior and binding studies of supersensitivity reviewed above, neuropsysiological studies with single-unit recording techniques were also undertaken to evaluate the hypothesis (Gallager et al., 1978).
Dopamine-containing cells in the zona compacta region of the substantia nigra were studied electrophysiologically following chronic haloperidol administration by both the direct iontophoresis of dopamine and the i.v. administration of graded doses of the dopamine agonist apomorphine. A two-fold increase in the sensitivity of dopamine cells to microiontophoretically applied dopamine, as well as significant increases in the sensitivity of these cells to i.v. apomorphine, was observed in rats chronically treated with haloperidol. However, animals treated with lithium administered in diet one week prior to and concurrently with i.p. haloperidol failed to show any increase in sensitivity to either iontophoretically applied dopamine or i.v. apomorphine. These results suggest that the dopamine-containing cells can be altered by chronic treatment with haloperidol and, in addition, that chronic lithium treatment appears to prevent this increase in sensitivity.
Thus, behavioral binding and electrophysiological evidence has been accumulated that lithium can prevent the development of supersensitive dopamine receptors in the central nervous system. It is possible that lithium's ability to prevent recurrent manic episodes may be related, at least in part, to its ability to stabilize dopamine receptor sensitivity. We have reviewed that a functional increase in dopamine may be involved in the manic process. Drugs that increase functional CSF dopamine, such as L-DOPA, may be associated with hypomania, and drugs that decrease functional dopamine, such as AMPT and pimozide, may be associated with a decrease in manic symptomatology.

REFERENCES

Angst, J., V. Autenrieth, F. Bram, M. Koukkou, H. Meyer, H.H. Stassen and U.Storck (1979). Preliminary results of treatment with beta-endorphin in depression. In Usdin, E., Bunney, W.E., Jr.and Kline, N.S. (ed.): Endorphins in Mental Research. MacMillan Press Ltd, New York,p.p. 518-528.
Ballenger, J.C. and R.M. Post (1978).Therapeutic effects of carbamazepine in affective illness. Commun. Psychopharmacol. 2, 159-175.
Ballenger, J.C. and R.M. Post (1980). Carbamazepine in manic-depressive illness: A new treatment. Am. J. Psychiatry 137, 782-790.
Brown, G. and S. Reichlin (1972). Psychologic and neural regulation of growth hormone secretion. Psychosom. Med. 34, 45-61.
Brown, W.A., R. Johnston, and D. Mayfield (1979). The 24-hour dexamethasone suppression test in a clinical setting: Relationship to diagnosis, symptoms and response to treatment. Am. J. Psychiatry 136, 543-547.
Bryson, R.W. and D.F. Martin (1954). 17-Ketosteroid excretion in a case of manic-depressive psychosis. Lancet 2, 365-367.
Bunney, W.E., Jr., E.L. Hartmann and J.W. Mason (1965a). Study of a patient with 48-hour manic-depressive cycles: II. Strong positive correlation between endocrine factors and manic defense patterns. Arch. Gen Psychiatry 12, 619-625.
Bunney, W.E., Jr., R.T. Kopanda, and D.L. Murphy (1977b). Sleep and behavioral changes possibly reflecting central receptor hypersensitivity following catecholamine synthesis inhibition in man. Acta Psychiatr. Scand. 56, 189-203.
Bunney, W.E., Jr., J.W. Mason, and D.A. Hamburg (1965b). Correlations between behavioral variables and urinary 17-hydroxycorticosteroids in depressed patients. Psychosom. Med. 27, 299-308.
Bunney, W.E., Jr., D.L. Murphy, F.K. Goodwin and G.F. Borge (1972). The "switch process" in manic-depressive illness. I. A systematic study of sequential behavioral changes. Arch. Gen Psychiatry 27, 295-302
Bunney, W.E., Jr., R.M. Post, A.E. Andersen, and R.T. Kopanda (1977a). A neuronal receptor sensitivity mechanism in affective illness (a review of evidence). Commun. Psychopharmacol. 1, 393-405.
Burt, D.R., I. Creese, and S.H. Snyder (1977). Anti-schizophrenic drugs: Chronic treatment elevates dopamine receptor binding in brain. Science 196, 326-328.
Carlsson, A. (1975). Receptor-mediated control of dopamine metabolism. In Usdin, E. and Bunney, W.E., Jr. (eds.). Pre-and Postsynaptic Receptors (Modern Pharmacology-Toxicology) Vol. 3, Marcel-Dekker, Inc., New York, pp. 231-236.
Carpenter, W.T., and W.E. Bunney. Jr. (1971). Diurnal rhythm of cortisol in mania. Arch. Gen. Psychiatry 25, 270-273.
Carroll, B.J. (1978). Neuroendocrine procedures for the diagnosis of depression. In Garattini, S. (Ed.). Depressive Disorders. Verlag, Stuttgard, pp. 231-236.
Carroll, B.J., and B. Davies (1970). Clinical associations of 2-hydroxycorticosteroid suppression and nonsuppression in serve depressive illness. Br. Med. J. 1, 789-791.
Carroll, B.J., J.F. Greden, M. Fernberg, N.McL. James, R.F. Hasket, M. Sterner, and J. Tarika (1980). Neuroendocrine dysfunction in genetic subtypes of primary unipolar depression. Psychiatry Res. 3, 251-258.
Casper, R.C., J.M. Davis, G.N. Pandey, D.L. Garver, and H. Dekirmenjian (1977). Neuroendocrine and amine studies in affective illness. Psychoneuroendocrinology 2, 105-113.
Corsini, G.U., M. Del Zompo, S. Manconi, C. Cianchetti, A. Mangoni and G.L. Gessa (1977). Sedative, hypnotic, and antipsychotic effects of low dose of apomorphine in man. In Costa, E. and Gessa, G.L. (Eds.). Nonstriatal Dopaminergic Neurons (Advances in Biochemical Pharmacology, Vol. 16. Raven Press, New York, pp.645-648.
Creese, I., D.R. Burt and S.H. Snyder (1977). Dopamine receptor binding enhancement accompanies lesion-induced behavioral supersensitivity. Science 197, 596-598.

Dalby, M.A. (1975). Behavioral effects of carbamazepine. In Penny, J.K. and Daly, D.D. (eds.). Complex Partial Seizures: Neurology Vol. 2. Raven Press, New York, pp. 331-343.
Davis, G.C., M.S. Buchsbaum and W.E. Bunney, Jr. (1979b). Analgesia to painful stimuli in affective illness. Am. J. Psychiatry 136, 1148-1151.
Davis, G.C., W.E. Bunney, Jr., M.S. Buchsbaum, E.G. DeFraites, W. Duncan, J.C. Gillin, D.P. van Kammen, J. Kleinman, D.L. Murphy, R.M. Post, V. Reus, and R.J. Wyatt (1979a). Use of narcotic antagonists to study the role of endorphins in normals and psychiatric patients. In Usdin, E., Bunney, W.E., Jr., and Kline, N. S. (Eds.). Endorphins in Mental Health Research. MacMillan Press Ltd, New York, pp. 393-406.
Davis, G.C., W.E. Bunney, Jr., E.G. DeFraites, J.E. Kleinman, D.P. van Kammen, R. M. Post and R.J. Wyatt (1977). Intravenous naloxone administration in schizophrenia and affective illness. Science 197, 74-77.
Davis, G.C., I. Extein, V.I. Reus, W. Hamilton, R.M. Post, F.K. Goodwin, and W.E. Bunney, Jr. Failure of naloxone to reduce manic symptoms. Am. J. Psychiatry, in press.
Ehrensing, R.H., A.J. Kastin, D.S. Schalch, H.G. Friesen, J. Vargas and A.N. Schally, (1974). Affective state and thyrotropin and prolactin responses after repeated injections of thyrotropin-releasing hormone in depressed patients. Am. J. Psychiatry 131, 6.
Emrich, H.M., C. Cording, S. Piree, A. Kolling, H.J. Moller, D. von Zerssen, and A. Herz (1979). Actions of naloxone in different types of psychoses. In Usdin, E., Bunney, W.E., Jr. and Kline, N.S. (Eds.). Endorphins in Mental Health Research. MacMillan Press Ltd, New York, pp 452-460.
Extein, I., A.L.C. Pottash, M.S. Gold, J. Cadet, D.R. Sweeney, R.K. Davies, and D.M. Martin (1980). The thyroid-stimulating hormone response to thyrotropin-releasing hormone in mania and bipolar depression. Psychiatry Res. 2, 199-204.
Fink, M., J. Simeon, T.M. Itil and A.M. Freedman (1970). Clinical antidepressant activity of cyclazocine, a narcotic antagonist. Clin. Pharmacol. Ther. 11, 41-48.
Gallager, D.W., A. Pert, and W.E. Bunney, Jr. (1978). Haloperidol-induced presynaptic dopamine supersensitivity is blocked by chronic lithium. Nature 273, 309-312.
Gerner, R.H., D.H. Carlin, D.A. Gorelick, K.K. Hui, and C.H. Li (1980). β-Endorphin: intravenous infusion causes behavioral change in psychiatric patients. Arch. Gen. Psychiatry 37, 642-647.
Gerner, R.H., R.M. Post, J.C. Gillin, and W.E. Bunney, Jr. (1979). Biological and behavioral effects of one nights sleep deprivation in depressed patients and normals. J. Psychiatry Res. 15, 21-40.
Gibbons, J.L. (1964). Cortisol secretion rate in depressive illness. Arch.Gen. Psychiatry 10, 572-575.
Gillin, J.C., R.M. Post, R.J. Wyatt, F.K. Goodwin, F. Snyder and W.E. Bunney, Jr. (1973). REM inhibitory effect of L-Dopa indusion during human sleep. Electroencephalogr. Clin. Neurophysiol. 35, 181-186.
Gold, P.W., F.K. Goodwin, T. Wehr, and R. Rebar (1977). Pituitary thyrotropin response to thyrotropin releasing hormone in affective illness: Relationship to spinal fluid amine metabolites. Am. J. Psychiatry 134, 9.
Gold, P.W., F.K. Goodwin, T.Wehr, R. Rebar and R. Sack (1975). Growth hormone and prolactin response to levodapa in affective illness. Lancet II, 1308-1309.
Gregoire, F., H. Brauman, R. deBuck, and J. Corvilain (1977). Hormone release in depressed patients before and after recovery. Psychoneuroendocrinology 2, 303-312.
Gruen, P.H., E.J. Sachar, N. Altman, and J. Sassin (1975). Growth hormone responses to hypoglycemia in postmenopausal depressed women. Arch. Gen Psychiatry 32, 31-33.
Hall, K.R.L. and E. Stride (1954). The varying response to pain in psychiatric disorders. A study in abnormal psychology. Br. J. Med. Psychol. 27, 48-60

Hartmann, E. (1968). Amitriptyline and Imiplamine: effects on human sleep. Psychophysiology 5, 207.
Hemphill, R.E., K.R.L. Hall and G.G. Crookes (1952). A preliminary report on fatigue and pain tolerance in depressive and psychoneurotic patients. J. Ment. Sci. 98, 433-440.
Janowsky, D.S., L.L. Judd, L. Huey, and D. Segal (1979). Effects of naloxone on normal, manic, and schizophrenic patients: Evidence for alleviation of manic symptoms. In Usdin, E., Bunney, W.E., Jr. and Kline, N.S. Endorphins in Mental Health Reseach. MacMillan Press Ltd., New York, pp.435-447.
Judd, L.L., D.S. Janowsky, D.S. Segal, and L.Y. Huey (1979). Naloxone-induced behavioral and physiological effects in normal and manic subjects. Arch. Gen. Psychiatry 37, 583-586.
Kirkegaard, C., N. Bjorum, and D. Cohen (1978). Thyrotropin-releasing hormone (TRH) stimulation test in manic-depressive illness. Arch. Gen. Psychiatry 35, 1017-1021.
Klawans, H.L. (1976). Read at Collegium Internationale Neuropsychopharmacologicum, Quebec City, Quebec.
Kline, N.S., C.H. Li, H.E. Lehmann, A. Lajtha, E. Laski, and T. Cooper (1977). Beta-endorphin-induced changes in schizophrenic and depressed patients. Arch. Gen Psychiatry 34, 1111-1113.
Kline, N.S., and H.E. Lehmann (1979). Preliminary results of treatment with beta-endorphin in depression. In Usdin, E., Bunney, W.E., Jr. and Kline, N.S. Endorphins in Mental Health Research. MacMillan Press Ltd, New York, pp. 500-517.
Kupfer, D.J., (1976). REM latency, a psychobiological marker for primary depressive disease. Biol. Psychiatry 11, 159-174.
Langer, G., G.Heinze, B. Reim, and N. Matussek (1976). Reduced growth hormone responses to amphetamine in "endogenous" depressive patients. Arch. Gen. Psychiatry 33, 1471-1475.
Lindstrom, L.H., E. Widerlow, L.M. Gunne, A. Wahlstrom and L. Terenius (1978). Endorphins in human cerebrospinal fluid: clinical correlations to some psychotic states. Acta Psychiatr. Scand. 57, 153-164.
Linnoila, M., B.A. Lamberg, G. Rosberg, S.L. Karonen, and M.G. Welen (1979). Thyroid hormones and TSH, prolactin and LH responses to repeated TRH and LRH injections in depressed patients. Acta Psychiatr. Scand. 59, 536-544.
Loosen, P.T., U. Merkel, and U. Amelung (1976). Combined sleep deprivation and chlorimipramine in primary depression. Lancet I, 156.
Maeda, K., Y. Kato, S. Ohgo et al. (1975). Growth hormone and prolactin release after injection of thyrotropin-releasing hormone in patients with depression. J. Clin. Endocrinol. Metab. 40, 501-505.
Martin, J. (1970). Neural regulation of growth hormone secretion. N. Engl. J. Med. 288, 1384-1393.
Matussek, N., M. Ackenheil, D. Athen. et al. (1974). Catecholamine metabolism under sleep deprivation of improved and not improved depressed patients. Pharmacopsychiatr. Neuropsychopharmacol. 7, 108-114.
Mendlewicz, J., P. Linkowski, L. Branchey, U. Weinberg, E.D. Weitzman, and M. Bronchey (1980). Abnormal 24-hour pattern of melatonin secretion in depression. Lancet II, 1362.
Merksey, H. (1965). The effect of chronic pain upon the response to noxious stimuli by psychiatric patients. J. Psychiatr. Res. 8, 405-419.
Muller, E.E., A. Pecile, M. Felici, and D. Cocchi (1970). Norepinephrine and dopamine injection into lateral brain ventricles of the rat and growth hormone relasing activity in hypothalamus and plasma. Endocrinology 86, 1376-1382.
Muller, P., and P. Seeman (1978). Brain neurotransmitter receptors after long-term haloperidol. Life Sci. 21, 1751-1758.
Murphy, D.L., H.K.H. Brodie, F.K. Goodwin, and W.E. Bunney, Jr. (1971). Regular induction of hypomania by L-DOPA in bipolar manic-depressive patients. Nature 229, 135-136.
Okuma, T., K. Inanaga, S. Otsuki, K. Sarai, R. Takahashi, H. Hazama, A. Mari, and

M. Watanabe (1979). Comparison of the antimanic efficacy of carbamazepine and chlorpromazine: A double-blind controlled study. Psychopharmacology 66, 211-217.
Okuma, T., A. Kishimoto, and K. Inoue (1975). Anti-manic and prophylactic effect of carbamazepine (Tegretol) on manic depressive psychosis. Seishin-Igaku 17, 617-630.
Okuma, T., A. Kishimoto, K. Inoue, H. Matsumato, A. Ogura, T. Matsushita, T. Naklao, and C. Ogura (1973). Antimanic and prophylactic effects of carbamazepine on manic-depressive psychosis. Folia Psychiatr. Neurol. Jpn. 27, 283-297
Pert, A., J.E. Rosenblatt, C. Sivit, C.B. Pert, and W.E. Bunney, Jr. (1978). Longterm treatment with lithium prevents the development of dopamine receptor supersensitivity. Science 201, 171-173.
Pflug, B. (1976). The effect of sleep deprivation on depressed patients. Acta Psychiatr. Scand. 53, 148-158.
Phillip, M., and C. Werner (1979). Prediction of lofepramine response in depression based on response to partial sleep deprivation. Pharmacopsychiatr. Neuropsychopharmakol. 12, 346-348.
Pickar, D., N.R. Culter, D. Naber, R.M. Post, C.B. Pert and W.E. Bunney, Jr., (1980) Plasma opioid activity in manic-depressive illness. Lancet I, 937
Pickar, D., G.C. Davis, S.C. Schulz, et al. Behavioral and biological effects of acute beta-endorphin injection in schizophrenic and depressed patients. Am. J. Psychiatry, In press.
Platman, S.R. and Fieve, R.R. (1968). Lithium carbonate and plasma cortisol response in affective disorders. Arch. Gen. Psychiatry 18, 519-594.
Post, R.M., R.H. Gerner, J.S. Carman, and W.E. Bunney, Jr. (1976). Effects of low doses of a dopamine-receptor stimulator in mania. Lancet I, 203-204.
Post, R.M., R.H. Gerner, J.S. Carman, J.C. Gillin, D.C. Jimerson, F.K. Goodwin, and W.E. Bunney, Jr. (1978). Effects of a dopamine agonist piribedil in depressed patients. Arch. Gen. Psychiatry 35, 609-615
Post, R.M., D.C. Jimerson, W.E. Bunney, Jr and F.K. Goodwin (1979). Dopamine and mania: Behavioral and biochemical effects of the dopamine receptor blocker pimozide. Psychopharmacology 67, 297-305.
Post, R.M., J. Kotin, and F.K. Goodwin (1976). Effects of sleep deprivation on mood and central amine metabolism in depressed patients. Arch. Gen. Psychiatry 33, 627-632.
Prange, A.J., I.C. Wilson, P.P. Lara et al. (1972). Effects of thyrotropin-releasing hormone in depression. Lancet 2, 999-1002.
Rechtschaffen, A., and L. Maron (1964). The effect of amphetamines on the sleep cycle. Electroencephalogr. Clin. Neurophysiol. 16, 438-445
Ritvo, E.R., E.M. Ornitz, S.La Franchi et al. (1967). Effects of imipramine on the sleep-dream cycle: an EEG study in boys. Electroencephalogr. Clin. Neurophysiol. 22, 465-468.
Rizzo, N.D., H.M. Fox, J.C. Laidlaw et al. (1954). Concurrent observations of behavior changes and of abrenocortical variations in a cyclothymic patient during a period of 12 months. Ann. Intern. Med. 41, 798-815.
Rotrosen, J.V. (1978). Neuroendocrine alterations in affective illness and schizophrenia. Read at Winter Conference on Brain Research, Keystone, Colorado.
Sachar, E.J., L. Hellman, D.K. Fukushima, and T.F. Gallagher (1970). Cortisol production in depressive illness: a clinical and biochemical clarification. Arch. Gen. Psychiatry 23, 289-298.
Sachar, E.J., L. Hellman, H. Roffwarg and F. Halpern (1973). Disrupted 24-hour patterns of cortisol secretion in psychotic depression. Arch. Gen. Psychiatry 28, 19-24.
Sachar, E.J., G. Mushrush, and M. Perlow (1972). Growth hormone responses to L-DOPA in depressed patients. Science 178, 1304-1305.
Sack, R.L., and F.K. Goodwin (1974). Inhibition of dopamine-β-hydroxylase in manic patients. Arch. Gen. Psychiatry 31, 649-654.
Schlesser, M., G. Winokur and B.M. Sherman (1979). Genetic sybtypes of unipolar primary depressive illness distinguished by hypothalamic-pituitary-adrenal axis

activity. Lancet 1, 739-741.
Schmocker, R. (1975). Experimentelle untersuchungen zur stabilitat des funklionssabilen geruslimplontates. Schweiz Monatsschr Zannheilkd 85, 154-163.
Schwartz, M., A.J. Mandell, R. Green et al. (1966). Mood, motility and 17-hydroxycorticoid excretion: a polyvariable case study. Br. J. Psychiatry 112, 149-156.
Shilgen, B. and R. Tolle (1980). Partial sleep deprivation as therapy for depression. Arch. Gen Psychiatry 37, 267-271.
Strombom, U. (1976). Catecholamine receptor agonists effects on motor activity and rate of tyrosine hydroxylation in mouse brain. Naunyn Schmiedebergs Arch. Pharmacol. 292, 167-176.
Takezaki, H. and M. Hanakoa (1971). The use of carbamazepine (Tegretol) in the control of manic-depressive psychosis and other manic-depressive state. Seishin-Igaku 13, 173-183.
Terenius, L., A. Wahlstrom, and H. Agren (1977). Naloxone (Narcan$^{(R)}$) treatment in depression: Clinical observations and effects on CSF endorphins and monoamine metabolites. Psychopharmacology 54, 31-33.
Toyoda, J. (1964). The effects of chlorpromazine and imipramine on the human nocturnal sleep electroencephalogram.Folia Psychiatr. Neurol. Japan 18, 198-221
van der Burg, W. and R.H. van den Hoofdakker (1975). Total sleep deprivation in endogenous depression. Arch. Gen. Psychiatry 32, 1121-1125.
Van Scheyen, J.D. (1977). Slaapdeprivatie bij de behandeling van unipolaire (endogene) vitale depressies. Ned T. Geneesk 121, 564.
Vogel, G.W. (1975). A review of REM sleep deprivation. Arch. Gen. Psychiatry 32, 749-761.
Vogel, G.W., A. Thurmond, P. Gibbons, K. Sloan, M. Boyd, and M. Walker (1975).REM sleep reduction effects on depression syndromes. Arch. Gen. Psychiatry 32, 765-777.
Von Knorring, L. (1975). The Experience of Pain in Patients with Depressive Disorders: Clinical and Experimental Study. Umea, Sweden, Umea University Medical Dissertations.
Voss, A. and H. Kind (1974). Ambulante behandlung endogener depression durch schlafentzug. Schweiz Rundsha. Med. 63, 564.
Wehr, T.A., A. Wirz-Justice, F.K. Goodwin, W. Duncan, and J.C. Gillin (1979). Phase advance of the circadian sleep-wake cycle as an antidepressant. Science 206, 710-713.
Woolf, P.D., R. Lantigua, and L.A. Lee (1979). Dopamine inhibition of stimulated growth hormone secretion: Evidence for dopaminergic modulation of insulin- and L-DOPA-induced growth hormone secretion in man. J. Clin. Endocrinol. Metal. 49, 326-330.
Wyatt, R.J., T.N. Chase, J. Scott, et al. (1970). Effect of L-DOPA on the sleep of man. Nature 228, 999-1000.
Wyatt, R.J., D.J. Kupfer, and J. Scott (1977). Longitudinal studies of the effect of monoamine oxidase inhibitors on sleep in man. Psychopharmacologia 15, 236-244.
Zis, A.P., R.W. Cowdry, T.A. Wehr, G. Muscettola, and F.K. Goodwin (1979). Tricyclic induced mania and MHPG excretion. Psychiatry Res. 1, 93-99.

Cellular Factors in Manic-depressive Illness: Blood and Brain

M. R. Issidorides

Department of Psychiatry, University of Athens, Eginition Hospital, Athens, Greece

ABSTRACT

A correlated study of locus coeruleus neurons from brain of suicide cases and of blood eosinophilic granulocytes from drug-free manic depressive patients revealed similar histochemical and ultrastructural alterations in their characteristic organoids, rich in basic proteins. These histone-like proteins, when free, are known to alter the permeability of cell membranes and to inhibit the response of cerebral tissue to electrical or other stimulation.

KEYWORDS

Locus coeruleus; suicide; manic depressive illness; spherical protein bodies; eosinophilic granules; major basic protein; membrane disruption; gigantocellular field of reticular formation (FTG).

INTRODUCTION

The depressive state, accompanied by the inherent tendency to self-destruction, often terminating in suicide, may be viewed as a dysfunction of the basic mechanisms of survival. These mechanisms are essential to the maintenance of life and have evolved from the adaptive modes that each species has found genetically advantageous in preserving its somatic and social integrity in its particular ecological environment. Although in man adaptive behavior for survival relies heavily upon social experience, which is processed by learning and memory, it is doubtful that a breakdown in this particular survival mechanism constitutes the substratum of suicide. The facts that a) the periodicity of the depressive state is independent of experiential cues, b) the core dysfunction is one of mood, and c) genetic components are implicated, clearly indicate the involvement of endogenous mechanisms of survival that ensure somatic integrity at the organismic level.

Among the endogenous survival mechanisms, probably the most relevant to affective illness is the mechanisms of sleep. Insomnia has been amply associated with depression (Zung, 1969) and has some value as a predictor of subsequent suicide (Rosen, 1976). In depressed patients REM latency is shortened (Kupfer, 1976). There is substantial evidence indicating that sleep deprivation (Pflug and Tölle, 1971), as well as REM sleep deprivation (Vogel and others, 1973) exercise a therapeutic effect on depression. In view of all this, the locus coeruleus (LC) of the pons emerged as the unavoidable target for study in the brain. Locus coerulus inactivity allows initiation of REM phenomena (Hobson, McCarley and Wyzinski, 1975). According to these authors, the decrease in locus coeruleus activity during REM is in phase with an increased activity in neurons of the gigantocellular field of the reticular formation (FTG). The reciprocal interaction of these two groups leads to cyclic REM episodes.

Although the neurons of the locus coerulus have been extensively studied by various approaches (Amaral, 1977), histochemical and ultrastructural studies in man are scarce and, as far as known, non-existent in patients. The design of the present cytological investigation derived from two different areas. Locus coeruleus neurons in man contain special spherical inclusions, rich in basic proteins which are markers of aminergic identity in the human brain (Issidorides and Panayotacopoulou, 1978). These "protein bodies" are decreased in LC neurons or absent from nigral neurons in Parkinsonism (Issidorides and others, 1978). On the other hand in a recent histochemical study of manic depressive patients (Issidorides and others, 1981) it was observed that the granules of blood eosinophils - also rich in basic proteins (Lewis and others, 1978) - were greatly disorganized in the drug-free patients. The purpose of the present investigation was to compare the histochemistry and ultrastructure of eosinophils with those of LC neurons, focusing on their basic proteins.

MATERIAL AND METHODS

Blood Study

The clinical material consisted of a group of 16 manic depressive patients who volunteered, after careful explanation of the procedure involved, for a longitudinal study of lithium prophylaxis, reported elsewhere (Issidorides and others, 1981). The age range of the patients was 21 to 69 years. The present study included 11 age-matched controls.

Brain Study

Human brains from suicide cases and from age-matched controls were obtained at autopsy and fixed in 10% formalin for the histochemical methods. Fresh-frozen brain tissues from suicide cases and matched controls for electron microscopy were obtained from the Human Specimen Bank, Wadsworth VA Hospital, Los Angeles. The entire sample studied included 25 control subjects with ages ranging from 20 to 85 years and 4 suicide cases aged 21, 22, 48 and 52 years. Causes of death in the control group were cardiovascular (15), traffic accidents (8) and bronchopneumonia (2). Causes of death in the suicide group were overdose of Valium, self-inflicted wounds, overdose of secobarbital with alcohol and hanging.

Methods

Light microscopy. Peripheral blood smears were fixed 2 hr after drying in 10% formalin and stained with Mallory's Trichrome method (Mallory, 1900) for basic proteins. This staining procedure includes the three acidic dyes, acid fuchsin, aniline blue and orange G. Paraffin sections from the medulla, pons and midbrain of the formalin-fixed brains were stained also with the above method. The stained preparations were photographed with color film (Agfachrome 50 L) and the color transparencies were printed in black and white for hightened contrast.

Electron microscopy. Fresh venous blood samples were obtained from patients and healthy controls using EDTA as anticoagulent. The erythrocytes were allowed to sediment at 37 °C for 3 hr and the leukocyte-rich plasma was collected and centrifuged at 250 g for 10 min. The supernatant was decanted and the leukocyte pellet was fixed with ice cold 2.5% glutaraldehyde (buffered with 0.2 M cacodylate, pH 7.2) for 45 min. The pellet was washed in buffer and processed further with potassium permanganate postfixation and phosphotungstic acid - hematoxylin block-staining as described in detail elsewhere (Issidorides and others, 1975). Thin sections were viewed in the EM without further staining.

RESULTS

Light Microscopy

The results of this study indicated that, following Mallory's Trichrome procedure, the staining reactions of "eosinophilic" granules in the blood granulocytes (Fig. 2) as well as of spherical protein bodies (PB) in aminergic neurons of the brain stem (Figs. 1,3) are identical, i.e. both types of organoids display red fuchsinophilia. This identity was confirmed by the parallel application in blood and brain (unpublished observations) of acidic dyes for basic proteins addressed to eosinophils.

The study of the control brains revealed that protein bodies in aminergic neurons, both in the perikaryon and in dendrites, are distinct, separate entities. This separateness was also true for the protein bodies in neurons of most aminergic cell groups of the suicide cases (Fig. 1), except for the neurons in the locus coeruleus. Figure 5 shows such a neuron displaying, in addition to melanin granules, a homogeneous mass of basic protein occupying half of the cell and containing agglutinated protein bodies (not too evident in this black and white version). The few, pale spherical bodies at the edge of the cell (Fig. 5, PB) suggested that the cytoplasmic basic protein may have diffused out from "leaky" protein bodies.

It is interesting to compare these findings with the morphology that prevails in the eosinophils of the drug-free patients (Fig. 4). Between and around the highly reactive, swollen nuclear lobes, the cytoplasmic area, free of granules was intensely fuchsinophilic while the few remaining granules,were paler than in the control of Fig. 2, and were agglutinated or fuzzy. These observations in drug-free patients showed, as previously reported (Issidorides and others, 1981), a loss of integrity of the granules in eosinophil leukocytes leading to diffusion of their basic protein into the cytoplasm.

At the level of light microscopy of blood and brain, changes in the eosinophils of drug-free manic depressive patients appeared to be a mirror image of cellular changes occurring in locus coeruleus neurons in the brains of suicide cases.

Electron Microscopy

The PTAH block-staining method, applied in this study, was originally developed to differentiate compact heterochromatin from loosely condensed chromatin and euchromatin fibers in blood leukocytes (Issidorides and others, 1975). Figure 6, showing a control eosinophil, demonstrates this differential nuclear staining: marginated compact heterochromatin is electron lucent (grey), while the small amount of euchromatin, at its inner border, facing the nucleoplasm, is electron-dense. Normal eosinophilic granules are known to contain a crystalloid core of arginine-rich protein, the so-called major basic protein (MBP), in a matrix segregating mainly myeloperoxidase, few other enzymes and macromolecules (Lewis and others, 1978). We observed that following PTAH block-staining these crystalloid cores revealed an ultrastructure similar to that of heterochromatin (Fig. 6).

As in the case of heterochromatin, the highly condensed state of the crystalloid core prevented the penetration of the large molecule of the acidic dye and the core, although very basic, remains electron lucent (grey) except for a thin peripheral band, which binds the stain. The matrix of the ovoid granules was finely fibrous, but otherwise unreactive after this method.

The spherical protein bodies in the neurons of the locus coeruleus in the control brains (Fig. 8) have also a heterochromatin-like ultrastructure after PTAH blockstaining, which emphasizes their compact state and corroborates their high concentration of basic proteins. (Issidorides and others, 1978). Further similarities of the neuronal protein bodies with heterochromatin and eosinophilic crystalloids were the thin peripheral, densely staining band surrrounding the electron lucent body, and the thin continuous limiting membrane (Fig. 8, arrow), which is usually separated from the protein body by a space.

The fine structure of the eosinophils of drug-free patients (Fig. 7) clarified the gross features observed in the histochemical staining of these blood cells. The few remaining ovoid granules were filled with densely staining fibrous material evidently deriving from "disolving" (decondensing) crystalloid cores. The area shown in the electron micrograph includes various stages of this dissolution, terminating in irregular masses of basic protein lying free in the cytoplasm (Fig. 7, arrowheads). These cells were further characterized by a coarse fibrous texture of the ground cytoplasm.

The fine structure of the protein bodies in the neurons of the locus coeruleus in brains of suicide cases (Fig. 9) dramatically justified the findings from light microscopy. Protein bodies of varying size and density were clustered together and occasionally agglutinated by twos or threes. The strong dye binding at their periphery revealed wide electron-dense band. All bodies showed a conspicuous lack of the thin limiting membrane. The electron-lucent central area was less lucent than in controls. A large number of agglutinated bodies displayed a dense central area. While individually membrane-less the granules, as a cluster,were surrounded by a very thin membrane (Fig. 9, arrow). These observations are interpreted as indicating a loss of integrity and separateness of the protein bodies in the suicide cases, probably, deriving from the absence of a limiting membrane and from the gradual decondensation of the compact structures.

At the level of electron microscopy of blood and brain, structural changes in the eosinophils of drug-free manic depressive patients and in the neurons of locus coeruleus in brains of suicide cases appear to have a common denominator. Namely, both display loss of integrity of their basic protein-rich organoids caused by decondensation and conformational changes of this protein as indicated by the altered dye binding. By disruption and absence, respectively, of the limiting membranes of these bodies the decondensed basic protein gains access to the cytoplasm.

DISCUSSION

The results of this study indicate that locus coeruleus neurons and blood eosinophils display related macromolecular changes in affective disorders. This finding is new, although the concept of blood elements (platelets) being used as peripheral equivalents of central nervous system structures (aminergic synaptosomes) is old. This correlated study of locus coeruleus neurons, from brain of suicide cases, and of blood eosinophils, from drug-free manic depressive patients revealed similar histochemical and ultrastructural alterations in their characteristic specific organoids. The major component of neuronal protein bodies is a basic histone-like protein (Issidorides and others, 1978). MBP, the major component of eosinophilic crystalloids, is a basic arginine-rich protein (Lewis and others, 1978). In this study both proteins, in their normal state and site were found secluded in distinct compact structures with a limiting membrane, and shared histochemical and ultrastructural characteristics with the heterochromatin. The significances of this finding is unclear at this stage. However, the observed mode of decompaction in the cells of the patients, suggestive of "euchromatization" or dissolution, has some bearing on important early work of McIlwain (1959). He found that under some natural and experimental conditions, cerebral arginine-rich histones, leaking from the nuclei to the cytoplasm, inhibit the response of cerebral tissue to electrical or other stimulation. He obtained the same effect from the application of exogenous histones and protamines to the slices. He pictures the histones as reaching a site involved in the cell's reaction to electrical pulses. On the other hand, MBP of eosinophilic granules, in addition to its involvement in tissue histamine metabolism (Archer and Jackas,1965), has been found to be neurotoxic to experimental animals when injected intracerebrally (Gordon, 1933). Probabaly, sharing the property of other "leaked" arginine-rich proteins, i.e. of altering the permeability of cell membrane (Fabriszewski and Rzeczycki, 1975), it may alter cellular functions.

In conclusion, the present findings from controls and patients are compatible with some structural instability prevailing in these normally compact, stable basic protein bodies and crystalloids. In the light of the cited literature, this instability may be relevant to the clinical data in manic depressive illness discussed in the introduction of this paper.

ACKNOWLEDGEMENT

Supported by grant No. 453/135 of the National Research Foundation of Greece.

LEGENDS

Fig. 1　　Human suicide. Neuron in gigantocellular field of pontine reticular formation. Protein bodies (PB) in soma and dendrites (arrowheads).

Fig. 2　　Eosinophil of control. Two nuclear lobes and granules.

Fig. 3　　Human control. Neuron of locus coeruleus. Protein bodies (PB) and scattered melanin granules.

Fig. 4　　Eosinophil of drug-free manic depressive patient. Swollen nuclear lobes, few granules, diffuse basic protein in cytoplasm.

Fig. 5　　Human suicide. Neuron of locus coeruleus with mass of basic protein and agglutinated protein bodies (PB).

Fig. 6　　Electron micrograph of eosinophil from control. Two nuclear lobes and ovoid granules containing crystalloid cores of arginine-rich protein (MBP).

Fig. 7　　Electron micrograph of eosinophil from drug-free manic depressive patient. Ovoid granules with crystalloid cores in various stages of decondensation. Basic protein diffused in granule space and free in cytoplasm (arrowheads).

Fig. 8　　Human control. Electron micrograph of locus coeruleus neuron showing membrane-bound (arrow) protein bodies and melanin granules (mg).

Fig. 9　　Human suicide. Electron micrograph of locus coeruleus neuron showing group of abnormal protein bodies: membrane-less, decondensed and agglutinated. Thin membrane (arrow) surrounds entire group.

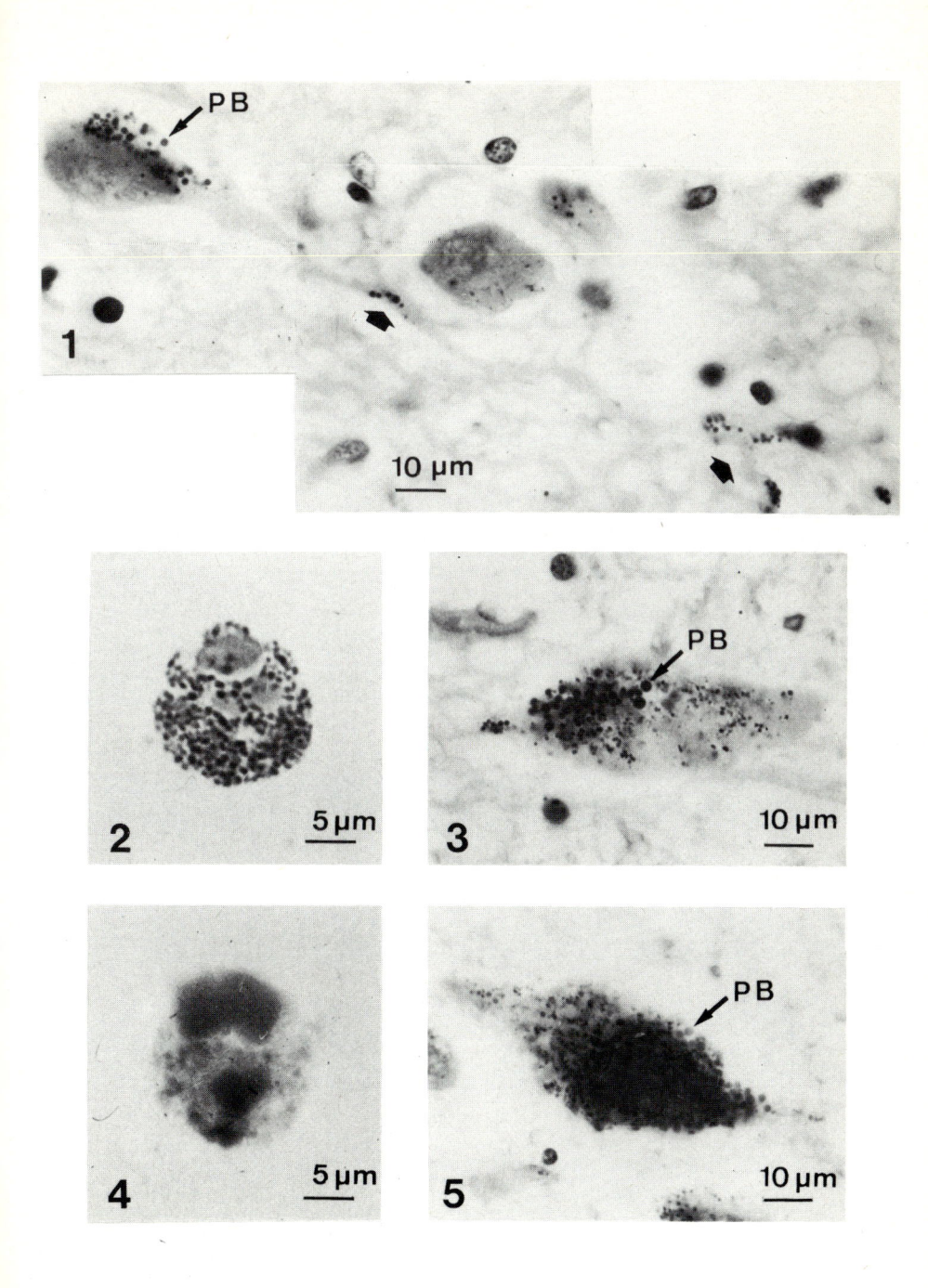

Cellular Factors in Manic Depressive Illness 105

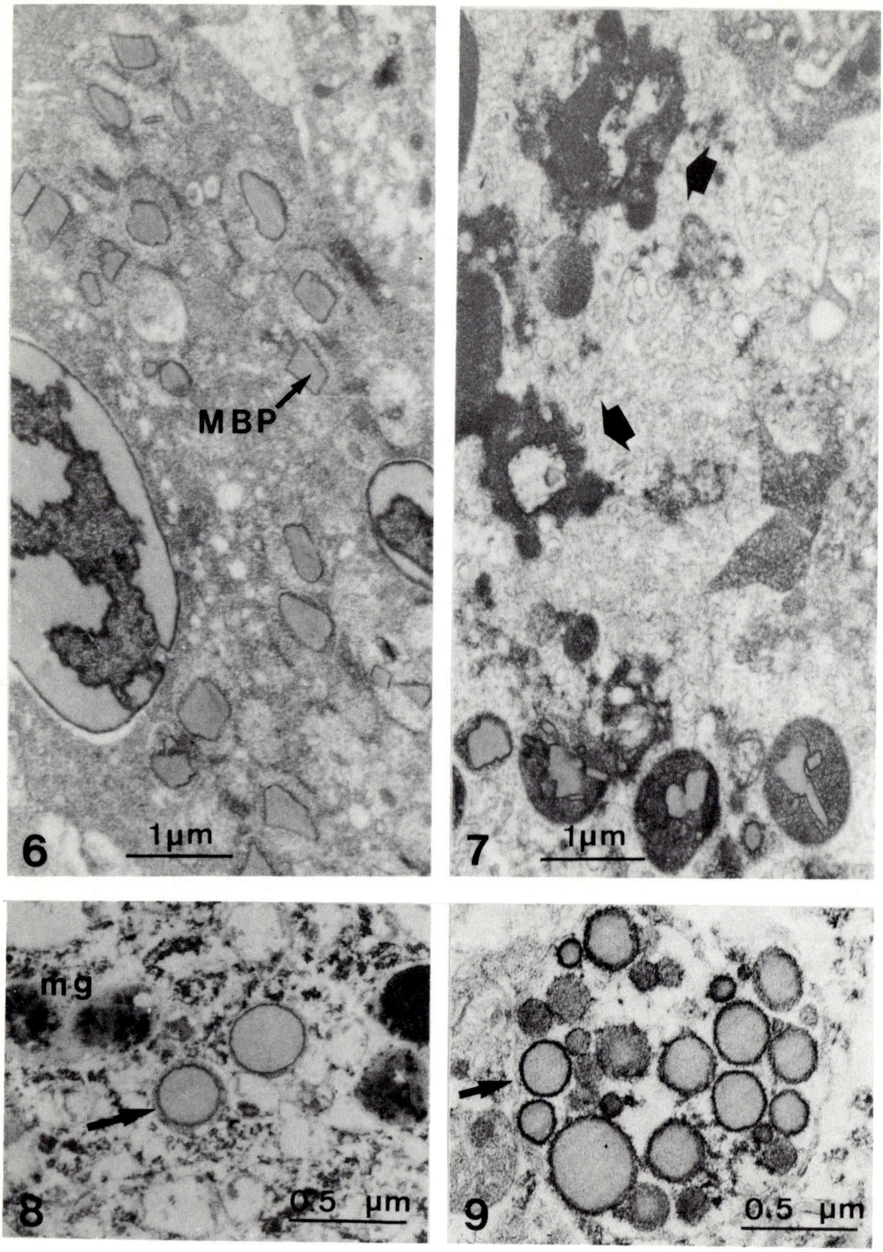
MBP
1μm
6
1μm
7
mg
0.5 μm
8
0.5 μm
9

REFERENCES

Amaral, D.G. (1977). Prog. Neurobiol., 9, 147-196.
Archer, G.T., and M. Jackus (1965). Nature (Lond), 205, 599-600.
Fabriszewski, R. and W. Rzeczycki (1975). Biochem. Biophys. Res. Commun., 65, 28-285.
Gordon, M.H. (1933). Br. Med. J., 1, 641-647.
Hobson, J.A., R.W. McCarley, and P.W. Wyzinski (1975). Science, 189, 55-58.
Issidorides, M.R., and M.T. Panayotacopoulou (1978). Neurosci. Lett. Suppl., 1, 270.
Issidorides, M.R., C.N. Stefanis, E. Varsou, and T. Katsorchis (1975). Nature (Lond), 258, 612-614.
Issidorides, M.R., C. Mytilineou, W.O. Whetsell, Jr., and M.D. Yahr (1978). Arch. Neurol., 35, 633-637.
Issidorides, M.R., E.P. Lykouras, G.N. Papadimitriou, M.T. Panayotacopoulou, and G.N. Christodoulou (1981). Bibliotheca psychiat., 160, 38-44.
Kupfer, D.J. (1976). Biol. Psychiat., 11, 159-174.
Lewis, D.M., J.C. Lewis, D.A. Loegering, and G.J. Gleich (1978). J. Cell Biol., 77, 702-713.
Mallory, F.B. (1900). J. exp. Med., 5, 15-20.
McIlwain, H. (1959). Biochem. J., 73, 514-521.
Pflug, B., and Tölle (1971). Int. J. Pharmacopsychiat., 6, 187-196.
Rosen, D.H. (1976). J. Am. med. Assoc., 235, 2105-2109.
Vogel, G.W., F.C. Thompson, Jr., A. Thurmond and B. Rivers (1973). The Effect of REM Deprivation on Depression. Karger, Basel. pp. 191-204.
Zung, W. (1969). Biol. Psychiat., 1, 283-297.

Clinical and Biological Correlates of a 48-hour Cycling Manic-depressive Patient

G. Trikkas, E. Varsou, E. Markianos, N. Karandreas and C. Stefanis

Department of Psychiatry, University of Athens, Eginition Hospital, Athens, Greece

ABSTRACT

This paper describes a manic-depressive patient, cycling on a 48-hour pattern of mood swings, with a rather unusual type of illness. Many clinical and biological parameters have been studied and some statistically significant findings between manic and depressed days were observed. These findings are discussed in relation to the observations of other authors.

KEYWORDS

Manic-depressive; rapid cyclers; switch process; 5HIAA, HVA, creatinine; c-AMP; MHPG.

INTRODUCTION

The study of patients with short-cycling periodic psychoses offers an unusual research opportunity for investigating the biological, behavioral and psychophysiological research mechanisms, underlying their psychiatric symptomatology. This study is particularly useful in elucidating the biological processes, that set in motion the switch mechanism from normality to abnormality and from one set of mental symptoms to another as the case is with bipolar affective disorders.
Menninger-Lerchenthal (1960) in his "Periodizität in der Psychopathologie" reported more than 64 cases of 48-hour cycling mental patients, mostly with organic psychoses.
Bunney and co-workers (1965a; 1965b), on the occasion of a patient with regular 48-hour manic depressive cycles, reviewed the litterature and found ten other similar cases, the first one been reported as early as 1804. Most of the reviewed cases were characterized as bipolars alternating from mania to depression and vice-versa. Interestingly enough in their majority these patients switched during the night while they were asleep.
Some additional cases of 48-hour cycling patients, who were subjected to a more detailed investigation, have been reported in the last decade (Jenner and co-workers,

1967, 1968; Bojanovsky, 1971; Hanna and co-workers, 1972: Kupfer and co-workers, 1972; Sitaram and co-workers, 1978; Gelenberg and co-workers, 1978; Doerr and co-workers, 1978; von Zerssen and co-workers, 1979; Paschalis and co-workers, 1980). The case to be presented is a manic-depressive female patient, who has all the typical features of a 48-hour cycler with very interesting course of her illness. The patient, while in the hospital, was subjected to a variety of clinical, psychological and laboratory tests throughout the period of hospitalization. From this study those findings that mainly indicate the differences in the clinical and biological profile of the patient during the alternating "depression" and "manic" days will be presented.

Case history

The patient, Mrs S., age 48 with a cyclothymic personality and pycnic body-type had no family history of affective disorders and had no complaints or symptoms of psychiatric significance until the age of 35. A few days after giving birth to her only child, she developed a typical anxiety-depressive episode. Following this, there were other depressive episodes each one lasting 20-30 days. In the course of 4 years she had 16 such episodes with a decreasing frequency. Subsequently the type of episodes had changed, each depressive episode being immediately followed by a short 10-20 days duration submanic or manic phase.
This pattern persisted for the last nine years and has changed to a 48-hour cycling pattern a short period prior to her admission to our hospital. Mania and depression alternated each other almost regularly every 24 hours with only occasional escapes, i.e., one 24 hour phase was followed by either a 24 hour normothymia or by extension of the preceding phase to the next day (phase doubling).
The switch from one phase to another took place consistently each morning between 10 and 10.30. The course of our patient's illness and change of pattern is illustrated in Fig. 1.

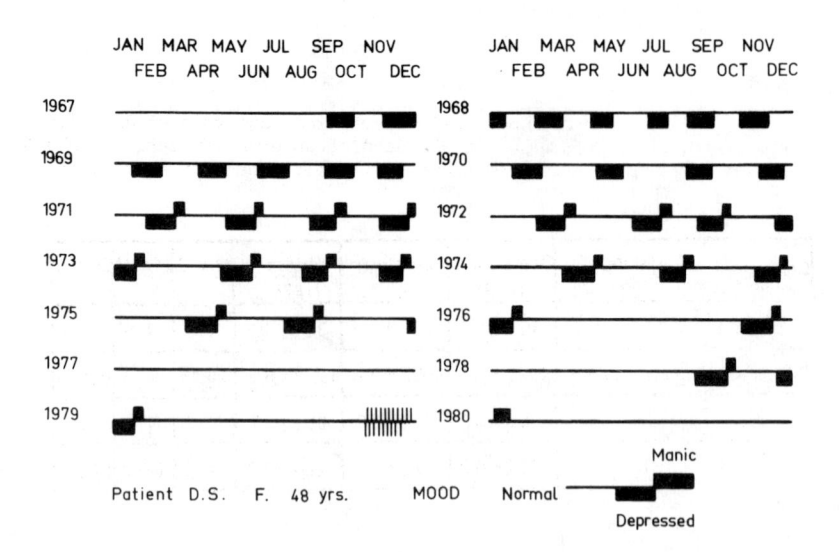

Fig. 1.

Clinical and Biological Correlates of a Manic-depressive Patient 111

Our patient had been hospitalized repeatedly in the past, mainly during her manic phase and was treated with neuroleptics. Antidepressant compounds were only occasionally administered, during the early depressive episodes of her illness. As will be discussed further, a few days after the spontaneous disruption of the 48-hour cycling, while the patient was in the hospital, she was given lithium bicarbonate and in one year's follow up no symptoms of affective disorder were observed.

METHOD

The study was carried out in a ward of the Psychiatric Clinic of the University of Athens, Eginition Hospital.
A routine laboratory investigation, during the first week of her hospitalization, failed to reveal any abnormality.
After a fortnight observation period, during which the patient was under the 48-hour cycle of mood swings, she was subjected to an intensive clinical and laboratory investigation.
Mood, systolic blood pressure (SBP), pulse and respiration rate (PR and RR) and temperature (T^o, by using centigrade thermometer in the axilla) were assessed five times per day (at 6 a.m., 10 a.m., 2 p.m., 6 p.m., and 10 p.m.). The patient's mood was evaluated by two experienced psychiatrists, using a seven point mood scale, +3 +2 +1 0 -1 -2 -3 (Jenner and co-workers, 1967). Our patient, while in the hospital, never slept during the day. Duration of night sleep was measured in hours by the nursing staff. Morning urine samples were collected during the study and 5-hydroxyindoloacetic acid (5HIAA), cyclic AMP (c-AMP), 3-methoxy-4-hydroxyphenylglycol (MHPG), homovanillic acid (HVA) and creatinine were determined. The concentrations of 5HIAA, c-AMP, MHPG and HVA in urine were expressed in μmol per gr creatinine. Diet and fluids were not controlled.
The entire observation period lasted three weeks. In the 8th and 10th days of the study two spontaneous total sleep deprivations of our patient occurred and since then the 48-hour cycle progressively lost its original pattern and Mrs S., became more or less normothymic. Morning urine findings were assessed as being related to mood state prevailing the previous day.

RESULTS

The mean values and the results from their statistical analysis of accumulated measurements of T^o, SBP, PR and RR for all days of observation during the depressive, manic and normothymic days are shown in Table 1. The N in this table repre-

Clinical parameters Ratings	Depressed N=34	Normal N=36	Manic N=25	M v D	M v N	D v N
Temperature (C°)	36.6±0.3	36.6±0.3	36.5±0.2	N.S.	N.S.	N.S.
Blood pressure (mmHg)	153.2±11.5	138.2±9.9	136.2±8.2	0.0005	N.S.	0.0005
Pulse rate (1')	84.1±6.8	87.2±5.7	85.5±5.7	N.S.	N.S.	0.05
Respiration rate (1')	28.2±6.3	22.6±3.7	26.2±3.8	N.S.	0.001	0.0005

Table 1

sents the total number of measurements per day for all days of observation. It is apparrent that SBP was significantly higher only during depression. PR was slightly elevated during depression compared to normothymia while R.R. was significantly elevated both during manic and depressive days. Temperature showed no significant differences.

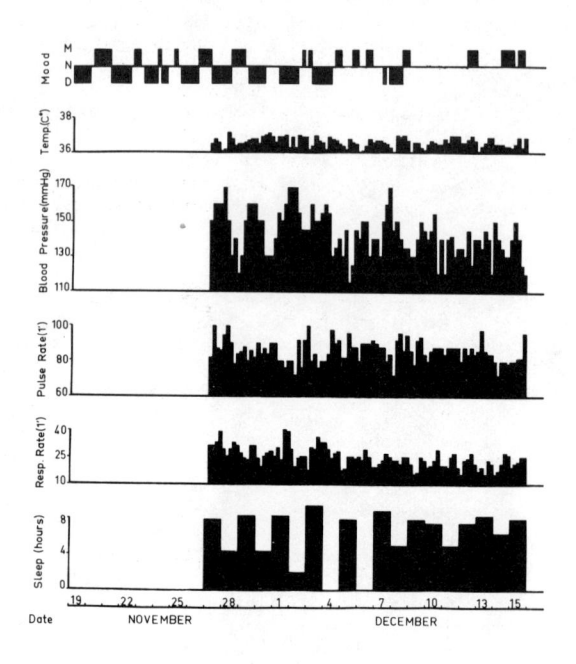

Fig. 2

In Fig. 2 the relationship of all these parameters to mood and night-sleep duration is illustrated; It is seen that our patient, while on depression during the day, slept only a few hours at night and had higher SBP and RR. Conversely, while on elated mood she slept more, had a lower SBP but the RR was as high as during depression.

Concentrations in morning urine (μmol/gCr)	Depressed N=5	Normal N=5	Manic N=7	D v N	D v M	N v M
c-AMP	3.0±0.6	3.0±0.4	3.5±0.9	N.S.	N.S.	0.02
MHPG	18.0±5.9	16.4±6.8	26.2±3.9	N.S.	0.006	0.02
HVA	12.2±0.9	16.3±5.0	17.4±5.8	0.01	0.03	N.S.
5HIAA	17.7±1.8	21.6±1.9	17.6±4.4	0.01	N.S.	0.03

Table 2

In Table 2 the results from measurments in morning urine of c-AMP, MHPG, HVA and 5-HIAA are shown. Comparative mean values for all depressed, normothymic and manic days, reveal slightly elevated cAMP during manic days, highly significant raise of MHPG during manic days, lowered concentrations of 5-HIAA during both manic and depressed days and finally lowered HVA concentrations during the depressed days. If we have a look at changes in time of these biological parameters (illustrated in Fig. 3), we may feel that we are sitting on thin ice, if we rely on the accumulated mean values of these parameters and try to associate them with the almost regularly alternating mood states during the period of our observation. As can be seen in this figure both total night-sleep durations and the morning urine investigated biological variables show a wave-form appearance, but they are not all in phase. Total night sleep duration urine volume and creatinine seem to have a day to day rhythmic variability, that is retained even when there is an occasional disruption in the 48-hour mood cycle. The other parameters (amine metabolites and cAMP) seem to be driven by slower and less regular pacemakers.

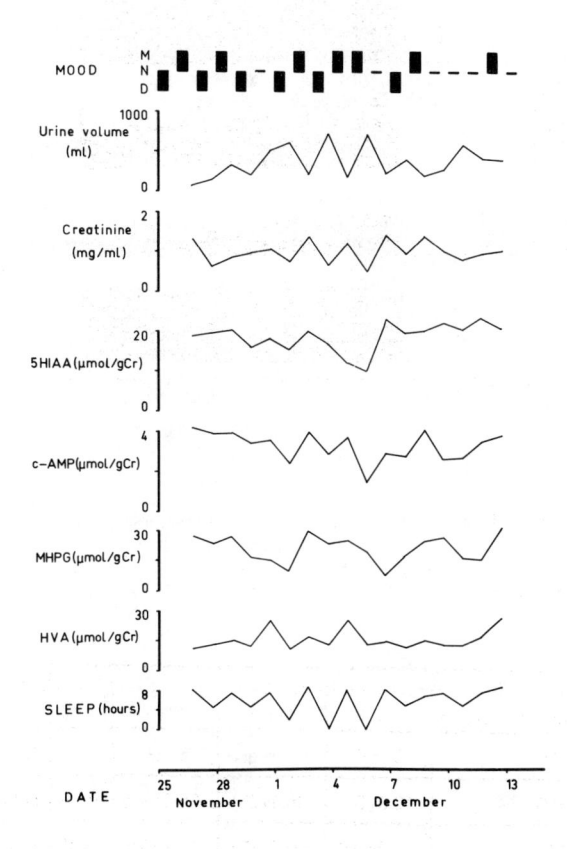

Fig. 3

DISCUSSION

One of the most interesting aspects of our case is the course of the illness. The

patient started as a unipolar and she had 16 reccurent episodes of depression in 4 years, before switching to bipolarity. This is important in view of clinical evidence, (Perris, 1966; Angst, 1966; Winokur and co-workers, 1969) strongly supported by recent neuroendocrinological findings (Carrol and co-workers, 1980a, 1980b) that unipolar and bipolar depression are distinct entities and strict criteria for separating the two should be applied.
The main of advocated criteria is that patients can only be diagnosed as unipolar depressives if they report three at least previous depressive episodes.
The number of episodes in our case far exceeded this limit and one might question the adequacy of this criteria for excluding masked bipolars from the group of unipolars. It is also to be noted that our patient had not but occasionally and only during the early period of her illness received tricyclic antidepressants. Thus, switching to bipolarity, cannot be considered a drug-induced phenomenon. While on the bipolar period of her illness,she usually was treated with neuroleptics either at hospital or home - in order to control the manic manifestations. Thus because of the treatment regime, we may consider the actual duration of depressive episodes as faithfully representing the natural duration determined by the illness process, but these may not be so for the manic phases, which were substantially modified by the neuroleptic treatment. Whether or not treatment with neuroleptics alone may have the same effect, that is postulated for antidepressants (Wehr and Goodwin 1979) in shortening the periods of out of phase biological rhythms and thus accelerate mood periodicity and ultimately lead to 48-hour cycling process, is an open question.
Most bipolars are treated with the two categories of drugs i.e. neuroleptics or antidepressants, and in some cases, with overlapping symptomatology, they are given synchronously. It would thus be of great clinical significance to know what the impact of these treatment schedules is on the long-term course of MD illness.

In most of the cases,thus far described in the literature,the switch was activated during the night while the patients were asleep (Jenner and co-workers, 1967; Bunney and co-workers,1965). In our case invariably it was activated in the morning several hours after awaking from the night's sleep. There are two points worth mentioning in this respect. The patient reports that the first manic episode was precipitated by a spontaneous total sleep deprivation, while she was in depression for several weeks. One night she could not fall asleep and the next morning she experienced for the first time an elated mood that soon escalated to a manic episode. This pattern persisted throughout the 9 year period of her bipolar illness; onset of depression-sudden total sleep deprivation-manic episode-normothymic interval-depression.
In addition to its other implications,regarding the relationship of sleep and mood switch mechanisms, this observation may indicate some usefullness of assessing mood reaction,following one night's total sleep deprivation in depressed patients,as a further means of separating true unipolars from "masked" bipolars. The other point, also relevant to the question of sleep and mood oscillations, is the observation that the 48-hour almost regular mood cycle showed initial signs of disruption and was finally terminated in one week following two (every other night) spontaneous sleep deprivations. Regarding the autonomic functions they have also shown significant correlations with alternating mood states although not as typically as sleep. Respiratory rate was significantly raised during both manic and depressive days, while pulse rate was only slightly changed and temperature showed no changes corresponding to mood states.
The findings from the morning urine measurements do not seem to provide a decisive clue regarding the biological mechanisms underlying the mood cycling.
MHPG concentrations were found to be significantly elevated during manic days. Other authors (Jones, 1971; Post and co-workers 1978) have found low MHPG concentrations in depressed days. This discrepancy might be more apparent than real. As shown in the Fig.2 the MHPG concentrations show a rythmic variability over the days of observation much lower than the circadian variation extending to an almost

double 48-hour cycle. Thus the variations in time of urine MHPG in itself may be of an established mood rhythmicity rather than to mood states. Provided that urimination rather than the comparative mean values between the depressed and manic days. Besides, as already shown by Wehr and Goodwin (1979), MHPG diurnal rhythms advances in phase during depression and in sigle per day measurments the MHPG values may reflect only phase changes.
The mean 5HIAA concentrations were found slightly lower in both depression and manic days compared to normothymic days. Jenner and co-workers (1967) also failed to see, in their own long studied 48-hour cycler, differences in 5HIAA urine concentrations during manic and depressed days. It is though to be remembered that contribution of central 5-HT turnover in urine 5-HIAA may be minimal and and of limited significance for interpreting CNS processes. Moreover, in our case, the difference in mean values may be accounted for by the profound drop of 5HIAA associated, at least in time, with the two spontaneous total sleep deprivations,that signalled the gradual desynchronization of the 48-hour cycle. The HVA concentrations were low during the depressed days compared to normothymic and manic days. These findings are at variance with those reported by Jenner and co-workers (1967) and somewhat in line with those reported by Bojanovsky (1971). It is noted though that differences in mean concentrations of urine HVA mainly derive from three sudden elevations, which concide with three deregulating events of the 48-hour cycle: the first one an escape, the second a double manic phase and the third, after a five days period of quiescence, the reemergence of a single isolated manic episode. This observation may suggest that HVA changes may be related to sudden disruption of an establishmed mood rhythmicity rather than to mood states. Provided that urine HVA concentrations reflect brain dopamine metabolism, a question still not definitively answered, one might interpret this finding as an additional support to the dopamine-controlled switch hypothesis of Bunney and co-workers (1970,1972).

Finally, as it has been pointed out, our patient, during the last period of her hospitalization, was given Lithium treatment and, in spite of the fact she was a rapid cycler, she improved, and for the last twelve months she is free of either depressive or manic episodes.

REFERENCES

Angst, J. (1966). Monogr. Neurol. Psychiat. 112, 1-118.
Bleuler, E.(1911). Dementia Praecox or the Group of Schizophrenias. Vienna (Trans. J. Zinkin 1950) Int. Univ. Press, New York.
Bojanovsky, J. (1971) Psychiat. Clin. 4, 336-346.
Bunney, Jr., W.E. and E.L. Hartmann (1965a) Arch. Gen. Psychiat., 12, 611-618.
Bunney, Jr. W.E., E.L. Hartmann and J.W. Mason (1965b). Arch. Gen. Psychiat. 12, 619-625.
Bunney,Jr. W.E., D.L. Murphy and F.K. Goodwin (1970). Lancet, I, 1022-1027.
Bunney, Jr. W.E., F.K. Goodwin, D.L. Murphy, K.M. House and E.K. Gordon (1972). Arch. Gen. Psychiat. 27, 304-309.
Carroll B.J., J.F. Greden and M. Feinberg (1980a) Lancet, 1, 321-322.
Carroll B.J., J.F. Greden and M. Feinberg (1980b) Psychiat. Res. 2, 251-258.
Cramer, J.C. (1959). Lancet 1, 1122-1126.
Doerr, P.,D. von Zerssen, M. Fischler and H. Schulz (1979). J. Affect. Disorders, I, 93-104.
Gelemberg, A.J., G.L. Klerman, E.L. Hartmann and P. Salt (1978). Br. J. Psychiat., 133, 123-129 .
Hanna, S.M., F.A. Jenner, I.B. Pearson, G.A. Samspon and E.A. Tompson (1972). Br. J. Psychiat., 121, 271-280.
Jenner, F.A., J.C. Goodwin, M. Sheridan, I.J. Tauber and M.C. Loban (1968). Br. J. Psychiat. 114, 215-224.
Jenner, F.A., L.R. Cjessing, J.R. Cox, A. Davis-Jones, R.P. Hullin and S.M. Hanna (1967) Br. J. Psychiat. 114, 895-910.

Jones de Leon, F., J.W. Maas, H. Dekirmenjian and J.A. Fawcett (1973). Science 179 300-302.
Kupfer, D.J., M. Bowers, G. Heninger and P. Mueller (1972). Psychophysiology 9,141
Menninger-Lerchenthal, E. (1960). Periodizität in der Psychopathology.Wilhelm Maudrich Verlag Wien - Bonn - Bern.
Paschalis, C., A. Pavlou and A. Papadimitriou (1980). Br. J. Psychiat., 137, 332-336.
Perris, C. (1966). Acta Psychiat. Scand. 42,(suppl 194) 1-188.
Post, R.M., F.J. Stoddard, C.J. Gillin, M.S. Buchsbaum, D.C. Runkle, K.E. Black and W.E. Bunney Jr. (1977). Arch. Gen. Psychiat. 34, 470-477.
Sitaram, N., J.N. Gillin and W.E. Bunney Jr. (1978). Biol. Psychiat., 13, 567-574.
Wehr, T.A., and F.K. Goodwin (1979). Arch. Gen. Psychiat., 36, 555-559.
Wever, R. (1975). Chronobiology 3, 19-55.
Wever, R. (1979). The Circadian System of Man. Springer, New York, Berlin, Heidelberg.
Winokur, G., P.J. Clayton and R. Reich (1969). Manic-Depressive Illness. C.V. Mosby Co, Medical Publishers, St. Louis.
Von Zerssen, D., R. Lund, P. Doerr, M. Fischler, H.M. Emrich and D. Ploog (1979). Neuropsychopharmacology. B. Saletu, E.D. Berner and L. Hollister, Pergamon Press, Oxford. pp. 233-245, New York.

Neuroendocrine Derangements in Depression

G. Tolis

Department of Medicine, McGill University, Royal Victoria Hospital, Montreal, Canada

ABSTRACT

During the last few years a variety of neuroendocrine abnormalities have been reported in depression. Thus, abnormalities have been described from almost every neuroendocrine system such as the hypothalamic-pituitary-adrenal (HPA), the hypothalamic-pituitary-thyroid (HPT), the hypothalamic-pituitary-gonadal (HPGn) etc. Some of them, like those pertaining to HPA axis, have been extensively studied, while only scarce data exists for others (i.e. these pertaining to HPGn axis). The neuroendocrine dysfunction in depression is thought to represent an alteration in the control of the hypophyseal function secondary to a functional uncoupling of the neurotransmitter-neuropeptide interaction.
Multivariate hormonal analyses may provide means for better diagnostic subclassification of depressive disorders and prove to be useful indices in assessing the therapeutic efficacy and predict the relapse of such patients.

KEY WORDS

Depression; neuroendocrine abnormalities.

INTRODUCTION

A number of disagreements exist regarding endocrine findings in depression. One reason for the discord is that affective disorders are characterised by heterogeneity with regard to nosology, physiopathology, and treatment. Besides this, the lack of uniformity in protocols among various investigators has resulted in discrepancies. Nevertheless, the literature is already enormous, and one must compliment the scientists for their innovative approaches to the biology of this mysterious mental disorder.

Hypothalamic-Pituitary-Thyroid axis
Interest in the endocrine glands, and in the thyroid as a key to mental disease arose in the last century. Emil Kraepelin was among the first to attempt to treat schizophrenia with thyroid extracts. Since then, numerous reports have appeared claiming or disclaiming the usefulness of thyroid hormones in the treatment of depressed patients.

We know that some depressed patients have improved after thyroid hormone administration. We do not know, however, whether those who improved were, in a broad sense, hypothyroid. It is possible that unsophisticated technology has resulted in erroneous diagnosis; it is also possible that some depressed patients, despite "normal" circulating hormone levels, needed higher concentrations of antidepressants in order to show a clinical response. In patients with peripheral resistance to thyroid hormones, the level needed to trigger physiological action exceeds the normal by many factors of magnitude. Even in instances of non-peripheral resistance we lack the refined techniques needed to establish the status of tissue-euthyroidism. The assessment of cardiac indices (e.g. systolic time interval), or hematological parameters (e.g. carbonic anydrase I of red blood cells), or neuromuscular status (e.g. muscle isoenzymes, half relaxation time of a tendon reflex) may provide this information.

The TRH test

At the moment, most investigators rely on the measurements of serum concentrations of thyrotropin (TSH), thyroxine (T_4), and triiodothyronine (T_3) to differentiate borderline hypo- or hyperthyroid status from normal. Other investigators, in addition, perform a TRH test which is expected to amplify the existing differences in patients with borderline nosology. Thus patients with exaggerated TSH response to TRH are thought to suffer biochemical hypothyroidism, whereas the reverse is true for hyperthyroidism.
Since the TRH test is commonly used in depressed patients for reasons not as yet clear, it may be wise to review the physiology behind this procedure. It is accepted today that the output of TSH from the anterior pituitary gland is governed by positive forces arising in the hypothalamus, and by negative signals arising in the brain and periphery. The thyroid hormones T_4 and T_3 exert a negative restraint on the TSH secreting pituitary cells ("long loop negative feed-back") (Vagenakis,1979). The tripeptide pyroglutamyl-proline-amide (TRH) is the only known peptidergic substance capable of enhancing TSH secretion. Recent studies have pointed out that a classical neurotransmitter (dopamine), a neuropeptide (somatostatin), and glucocorticoids can all suppress TSH secretion under both basal and provoked conditions (that is, after administration of TRH). A normal response to TRH is characterized by a three-fold or larger increment of serum TSH occuring within 30 minutes of the TRH injection. (Basal serum TSH, T_4, and T_3 should be normal at the beginning of the test; otherwise, the interpretation of the data is problematic. For example, if serum T_4 and T_3 are elevated, and no response to TRH is seen, this should not be interpreted as pathological but as a sign of physiological negative feedback restraint, caused by hyperthyroidism). If, in the presence of normal thyroid hormones, there is no response to TRH, or only a diminished response, then two hypotheses can be offered as explanation.Either the patients is relatively hyperthyroidic, or there is an excess of factors suppressing TSH release. The latter possibility is difficult to establish with the exception of coexisting Cushing's syndrome or the intake of large amounts of glucocorticoids (e.g. prednisone for rheumatoid arthritis).
In affective disorders, TSH release after TRH may be decreased, normal, or increased. This wide range of response is seen particularly if neurotic depressives, alcoholics, manic depressives, and unipolar depressives are all grouped together (Ehrensing and co-workers, 1974; Amsterdam and co-workers, 1979; Mendlewicz and co-workers, 1979a; Asnis and co-workers, 1980; Extein and co-workers, 1980; Kirkegaard and Bjorum, 1980; Loosen and Prange, 1980; Weisenburger and co-workers, 1980). Most investigators agree, however, that in unipolar depression, there is blunted TSH response to TRH (Asnis and co-workers, 1980;). Following treatment of the depressive disorder there may be normalisation of the response or there may be no change whatsoever (Asnis and co-workers, 1980; Kirkegaard and Bjorum, 1980). That the absence of improvement in TSH response to TRH is predictive of future re-

lapse is still debatable (Asnis and co-workers, 1980; Extein and co-workers, 1980; Kirkegaard and Bjorum,1980).

TRH as therapeutic agent

TRH has been administered for therapeutic as well as diagnostic purposes. It was used as a result of earlier data showing a beneficiary effect of thyroid hormones or thyrotopin in some patients with depression. Following initial enthusiastic reports (Prange and Wilson,1972; Chazot,1974), independent researchers were unable to confirm a beneficial effect of TRH in depression (Takahashi and co-workers,1973; Hollister and co-workers,1975). In a recent, careful study, however, it was shown that in a small number of patients TRH did have some salutary effect; this effect, however, was less impressive than that of amitryptylline and it was inversely related tothe status of thyroid economy (Karlberg and c0-workers,1978). More such studies are needed; they may shed some light on early reports describing an effect of thyroid extracts in some if not all patients.
It may indeed be the case that patients showing improvement had subclinical hypothyroidism. Other hypotheses have also been formulated in an attempt to explain the efficacy of TRH in the treatment of depressive disorders. However, the view that there is an endogenous TRH deficiency in depressive disorders is nontenable because patients with hypothalamic TRH deficiency show a normal, if not exaggerated response to TRH, and have concomittant hypothyroidism.
The mechanism whereby TRH improves depression is unknown. Unquestionably TRH has effects upon the central nervous system which are independent of those of TSH and thyroid hormones. It produces characteristic electroengephalographic complexes. It alters the effects of barbiturate and ethanol effects on arousal. It modifies the efficacy of other small neuropeptide or transmitters or CNS-acting substances (Renaud and co-workers,1978).
In summary, TRH has been used both as a diagnostic tool and as a therapeutic treatment in patients with severe unipolar depression. As mentioned earlier, on the basis of the available data it is impossible to explain the blunted TSH response to TRH. Studies of the concomittant activity of the hypothalamic pituitary adrenal (HPA) axis would be required to discern cortisol overproduction. Measurements of growth hormone responses to provocative stimuli may help identify an increased somatostatin output. Were somatostatin output increased, both GH and TSH release would be diminished. (It should be noted, however, that this diminuation may also be seen in hypercortisolemic states, for instance in Cushing's syndrome).
Finally, in order to assess whether the decreased TSH release is due to excess dopaminergic tone, the following parameters should be employed during testing. First, the prolactin relase to TRH should be decreased. Second, the GH response to any provocative test should be intact or exaggerated.Third, a reversal of the TSH suppressibility should be accomplished by a short treatment of antidopaminergic medications. Undoubtedly the standardisation of the TRH test protocol and the concomittant evaluation of the factors already mentioned may add to the further understanding of the role of TRH and thyroid hormones.

Hypothalamic-Pituitary-Adrenal axis

Emotional and behavioral changes are known to occur in patients with adrenal disorders, e.g. with Addison's disease or Cushing's syndrome. In fact, the psychiatric presentation of some patients with Cushing's syndrome is occasionally the presenting feature, and it may be dramatic. Studies of the hypothalamic-pituitary-adrenal axis (HPA) axis in depressed patients reveal a constellation of biochemical data could be compatible with adrenal hyperfunction.
Under normal circumstances there is a circadian rhythm in the pulsatile secretory pattern of ACTH and cortisol. Nadir values are reached by midnight unless there is

a sleep reversal (as is the case, for instance, with night guards). From the pituitary ACTH is released in episodic bursts, presumably because the ACTH releasing factor arrives at the hypophysial cells in an episodic manner. ACTH release seems to be affected by glucocorticoids and a variety of neurotransmitters. Serotonin is believed to promote ACTH secretion since administration of antiserotonergic drugs (e.g. cyproheptadine) attenuates its release. Yet the role of serotonin and other neurotransmitters in the release of ACTH in relation to stress, sleep, or episodic pattern is unknown.
Glucocorticoids, and in particular cortisol, exert a negative, suppressive effect upon ACTH release as a result of their effect upon the anterior pituitary. Dopamine or dopamine agonist drugs, somatostatin, and the opiate receptor blocking agents have all been reported to suppress ACTH secretion in some pathological circumstances, but their role in the physiological control of ACTH is unknown.

In an appreciable number of depressed patients, the following abnormalities of the HPA axis have been reported (Carroll and Mendels, 1976a):
1. Increased cortisol production rate.
2. Increased number of secretory spikes throughout the 24-hour period.
3. Preservation of the circadian rhythm, in spite of a "shift to the left".
4. Elevated plasma and cerebrospinal fluid cortisol.
5. Decreased stimulability of the pituitary corticotropes to hypoglycemia.
6. Decreased suppressibility to dexamethasone.

It should be pointed out that not all the above abnormalities can be demonstrated in all depressed patients. As a matter of fact, as many as 50 per cent of patients with depression may not have a demonstrable abnormality of the HPA axis. However, that demonstration of abnormal HPA axis may be of value in supporting the diagnosis of endogenous depression (Carroll and Mendels, 1976b).

The Dexamethasone Test

The dexamethasone test is easily performed, it causes little inconvenience to the patient but it is, as yet, unstandardized. Accordingly, there have been problems. Earlier investigations claimed the plasma cortisol suppressed normally to dexamethasone. Studies showing suppression, however, exhibited several defects: the researchers used the 8 a.m. plasma cortisol as an index of suppressibility and they administered only 1 mg of dexamethasone. In subsequent studies, in which 2 mg of drug were used, and measurements of plasma cortisol were made at 8 a.m., 4 p.m., and 11 p.m. the next day, it became obvious that as many as half the patients with severe endogenomorphic depression showed as escape phenomenon (Carroll and Mendels, 1976a; Carroll and Mendels, 1976b; Brown and co-workers, 1979; Schlesser and co-workers, 1979).
Although the 8 a.m. values were suppressed, the subsequent values were higher than those of controls, or patients with schizophrenia or depressive neurosis.

Similarly, the 24 hour urinary output of cortisol following dexamethasone was lower in the controls than in depressed patients. Of particular interest was the observation that the majority of depressed patients who exhibited the above abnormalities had higher midnight plasma cortisol values, although a circadian rhythm was preserved. These findings have been confirmed in studies involving close to 400 patients. The explanation of the non-suppressibility is not known. Equally mysterious, moreover, is the fact that a large group of patients with depression will suppress. Is the dexamethasone test therefore a useful tool?
A recent study indicated that although there is no difference between "suppressors" and "non-suppressors" with regard to previous episodes, family history, symptoms, or medication intake, the "non-suppresors" tend to have more severe depression and to respond better to anti-depressants than do suppressors (Brown and co-workers, 1979). Similary, other investigators have classified depressed patients according

to the level of neurotransmitter metabolites in urine; they have also found that on this basis they can predict response to antidepressant medication (DeLeon - Jones and co-workers, 1975).Unfortunately, large studies concomittantly assessing the HPA axis and metabolites of catecholamines or serotonin have not been reported. The hypothesis developed at present with regard to non-suppressibility is that during the acute phase the tone of the limbic system is disturbed or "upregulated". Although the analysis of the suppressibility of the HPA axis following administration of dexamethasone reveals an abnormality in a large percentage of patients, the use of provocative tests for cortisol secretion is of questionable significance in characterizing these patients. Certainly the adrenal response to ACTH is comparable to normal among all subclasses of depressed patients. When insulin-induced hypoglycemia is used, the cortisol responses elicited cover a wide spectrum from poor to exaggerated (Mueller and co-workers,1969;Sachar and co-workers,1971; Perez-Reyes,1972;Endo and co-workers,1974).The smallest increments have been reported in association with basal elevation of plasma cortisol and poor suppressibility (Carroll,1969).
In such patients a disturbance in the circadian cortisol rhythm can also be demonstrated if properly assessed. Thus, the circadian rhythm in depressed individuals is preserved when judged on the basis of 8 a.m. and 11 p.m. cortisol values; the episodic bursts of plasma cortisol, however, as compared to control subjects, are enhanced during late evening hours. That this finding probably reflects a disturbance in the limbic system structures involved in ACTH control, and is not a response to specific stress, is suggested by studies showing that during acute stress patients with phobic neurosis show no comparable disturbance of the circadian profile.
In summary, endogenomorphic depression creates a spectrum of disturbance of the HPA axis. These disturbances may be mild in early stages of the condition, consisting simply of elevated cortisol production during daytime. They may be moderate, consisting of elevation of cortisol secretion during both day and night. The suppressibility will be apparent at 8.a.m. after the midnight,administration of dexamethasone. More severe disturbances entail escape to suppression as early as 8 hours after administration of 2 mg of dexamethasone.
Most of these derangements resemble diencephalic Cushing's syndrome (Gold,1980). Since it has recently been learned that in Cushing's syndrome TRH or naloxone will paradoxically stimulate or suppress ACTH release (Tolis and co-workers,1979a), and that long-term improvement can be achieved with the use of antiserotonergic or dopamine receptor agonists, it may be worthwhile to apply the strategies derived from Cushing's studies to patients with depression. Investigations of this sort might give us a better functional neuroendocrine subclassification of patient with depressive disorders and provide us with guidelines for better evaluation of the efficacy of the various antidepressant medications.

Hypothalamic pituitary gonadal axis
A.Females

The HPGA activity depends on numerous variables (Naftolin and Tolis, 1978). Its normality is expressed in the female by the occurence of cyclic changes in the endometrial activity manifested by monthly vaginal bleeding. Biochemically, the period between bleedings is divided into three phases: the follicular, the periovulatory, and the luteal. At midcycle there is a surge in serum LH and FSH due to hypothalamic release of LHRH, and increased gonadotrope sensitivity. This LH peak can be blocked by antibodies to LHRH or drugs that affect the availability of monoamines. These are believed to trigger LHRH release. Sex steroids,adiposity,melatonin, prolactin, and endogenous opiates are among the factors already studied which can modulate negatively the activity of the hypothalamic-pituitary circuit (Naftolin and Tolis,1978; Yen,1980).
The ability of the pituitary gonadotropes to release gonadotropin is tested by administering LHRH and recording plasma changes in LH and FSH. Controversy exists

regarding the amount and the mode of administration of LHRH. The injection of LHRH in a bolus provides one peak, whereas infusion induces two spikes of LH release thought to represent different gonadotropin pools. Doses of 10, 25, and 100 μg all have quantitatively different effects on LH release. We still do not know, however, whether these changes are physiological or pharmacological in origin. And in contrast to LHRH, which provokes LH release when given in a single bolus, a neurotransmitter, dopamine, seems to inhibit pituitary gonadotropin ralease; whether this represents only pharmacology (for the human at least) is also unknown.
Activation of the hypothalamic sector of the module can be achieved by the administration of estrogens and clomiphene in normal subjects. The former is thought to detect the status of the positive and the latter the status of the negative feedback control of gonadotropin secretion.
Women who suffer severe weight loss (more than 20 per cent of ideal body weight), or who have pituitary tumors (with or without hyperprolactinemia), or isolated gonadotropin deficiency, or women who are treated with birth controll pills, all will show distorted responses to LHRH and will practically always have no response to estrogens or clomiphene.
Our studies in amenorrheic depressed women without weight loss show that there is hypoestrogenism, normal or low gonadotropin output, preservation of the responses to LHRH but absence of responsiveness to estrogens or antiestrogens (Tolis, 1981). These findings point to a suprahypophyseal defect, similar to that detectable in women with anorexia nervosa. In support of a central disorder are the observations of decreased LH output in depressed menopausal patients (Altman and co-workers,1975) and the ability of drugs (preventing availability of monoamines to LHRH neurons) to inhibit the expected LH rise post-gonadectomy in the experimental animal (Ojeida and McCann, 1974). We must investigate further whether there is excess dopaminergic or endorphinergic tone (thought to suppress LHRH release) in amenorrheic women with depression. To do this, studies are required employing drugs that block dopamine and endorphin receptors. Such protocols have already been exploited for the study of hypothalmic anovulatory syndromes (Ojeida and McCann, 1974).

B.Males
Males with depression often complain of impotence. If impotence is associated with decreased libido, then investigations are needed to exclude other metabolic-endocrine disorders like uremia, liver failure, or putuitary tumors (Tolis and co-workers,1973; Tolis and co-workers,1980). If measurements of prolactin, gonadotropins, and sex steroids are normal, then monitoring of the nocturnal penile tumescence may differentiate between psychogenic and organic impotence (Fisher and co-workers, 1979). Reported studies in depressive disorders are scarce. According to the few that do exist, although the pituitary gonadotrope ability to release LH as tested with bolus LHRH administration is preserved, there appears to be some difference in various types of the disease. Of potential diagnostic and therapeutic interest is the reported paradoxical LH release to dopamine in manic patients (Gold and co-workers,1980). If one accepts that libido is heightened in mania (Gold and co-workers,1980) and that dopamine agonists or precursors (bromocriptine or levodopa) can enhance sexual activity in certain patients, i.e. those with Parkinson's disease, studies of the HPGA with the above-mentioned techniques might serve as a guide for further therapeutic attempts. Whether these neurotransmitter-like drugs have a direct effect upon sexual behaviour, or whether it is mediated via changes of LHRH prolactin or endogenous opiates is remains to be tested (Moss and McCann,1975;Tolis and co-workers,1978;Gessa and co-workers,1980;Gold and co-workers,1980).

Growth hormone

Growth hormone (GH) is secreted from the anterior pituitary gland throughout life. Metabolic and neuronal factors influence its secretory pattern. It is believed that somatostatin is a major regulatory peptide; it works in concert with peripheral growth hormone dependent (i.e.somatomedins), or independent growth factors to provide an inhibitiry tone on the anterior pituitary somatotropes. Typically,in provide an inhibitory tone on the anterior pituitary somatotropes. Typically, in severe malnutrition, when somatomedin peptides are not synthesized in normal quantities, levels of fasting GH are elevated. This should be taken into account when analysing serum GH levels in depressed patients who have shown long-term abstinence from food, or who suffer from maltutrition. A decline in fasting serum GH after refeeding has been noted by many investigators studying various pathological circumstances, including anorexia nervosa.

Growth hormone production can be stimulated by exercise, ingestion of certain aminoacids, deep sleep, and administration of various pharmacological agents, including dopamine, apomorphine, bromocriptine, clonidine,5-OH-tryptophan, and the endogenous opiates-endorphins and enkephalins (Martin, 1979). Such data are taken to indicate that dopaminergic, noradrenergic, serotoninergic, and opiergic receptors are involved in the control of GH secretion. The mechanism whereby these agents stimulate GH secretion is not completely understood. It is presumed that these factors either suppress somatostatin release or stimulate the secretion of an independent growth-hormone releasing factor whose chemical identity is still unknown.

In patients with endogenomophic unipolar depression, the GH release mechanism is apparently impaired (Gruen and co-workers, 1975; Brown and co-workers, 1978). It should be mentioned, however, that earlier data showing a decreased GH response to levodopa apomorphin and 5-hydroxytryptophan have been criticized for lack of proper controls. Along these lines, we might mention that also in need of standardization is insulin-induced hypoglycemia as a test. The percent of blood sugar drop and the achievement of a certain absolute level should be set as prerequisites which must be met before test results are considered unquestionable (Mueller and co-workers, 1969, Brown and co-workers, 1978).

The rise in serum GH following administration of certain pharmacological agents seems to be significantly decreased as compared to normal subjects matched for age, or as compared to patients with neurotic depression. Although the mechanism is unknown, the decrease in plasma norepinephrine levels and urinary MHPG excretion in those patients showing decreased responsiveness may suggest the existence of a defective noradrenergic status in depression (Matussek, 1977). In contrast to the inability of clonidine, hypoglycemia, or even amphetamine to induce a normal GH response, levodopa seems capable of so doing (Sachar, 1974). This may suggest a selective alteration in noradrenergic but not dopaminergic status in unipolar depression. Recovery from the depressive state may be associated with reversibility of this abnormality in GH release in most patients. Whether a persistent abnormality in GH release can predict a relapse has not been critically evaluated.

In order to avoid interpreting as physiology data obtained with the use of pharmacological agents, various attempts have been made to use a physiological stimulus for GH release. One stimulus chosen was sleep. Although original reports confirmed a reduced GH release during sleep (Sachar, 1973), the conclusions were invalidated, partly because the sleep was abnormal (Snyder, 1968).

More recently, in an effort to explore the GH dynamics in depression, studies have been done which showed a paradoxical GH rise after TRH (Chazot, 1974; Maeda and co-workers, 1975). Similar paradoxical responses have been described in patients with malnutrition, anorexia nervosa, hypothyroidism, and acromegaly; they are taken to imply an alteration in the GH receptor of the somatotropes (Tolis and co-workers, 1979b). The demonstration of increased GH release to TRH tends to exlude an increased somatostatinergic tone in depression, a theory proposed by some investigators to explain reduced GH responses following insulin-induced hypoglycemia.

In summary, the most consistent finding in unipolar depression is the reduced GH response to insulin-induced hypoglycemia, and possibly to clonidine. Studies are

RAD - F

needed to evaluate GH responses in depressed patients to other provocative procedures like sleep, administration of dopamine receptor agonists, and 5-OH tryptophan. In addition, follow-up studies of the various response patterns during treatment are required if we are to choose suitable pharmacological agents and to identify those patients who may relapse, if treatment is prematurely discontinued.

Prolactin

The introduction of reliable immunoassay methods has facilitated the study of prolactin (PRL) dynamics in health and disease (Tolis and Francs, 1979). It is believed today that PRL secretion from the anterior pituitary is controlled by the hypothalamus. Substances which inhibit its secretion collectively are called prolactin inhibitory factors (PIFs). Substances which enhance it are called prolactin releasing factors (PRFs). The sequence of a specific peptidergic PRF pf PIF is unknown (Tolis and Francs, 1979).

The maintenance of normal serum PRL is established by tonic inhibitory control. This control is exerted primarily by dopamine; serotonin, and endogenous opioid peptides seem to enhance PRL secretion in animal and man. Of the three sequenced hypothalamic factors, SRIF, GnRH, and TRH, only the latter provokes PRL secretion. Yet TRH is not the only prolactin-releasing factor. Estrogens enhance PRL secretion in the experimental animal and man. Changes in circulating thyroid hormone levels also modify prolactin secretion (Tolis and Francs, 1979).

A circadian rhythm for serum PRL seems to exist, but it is less well defined than that of ACTH. There is also a sleep-related increase in serum PRL that is independent of the sleep-induced GH changes (Tolis, 1980). Stress, labyrinthic stimulation, amygdalar stimulation, and generalised epilepsy all have been reported to increase following prolactin discharges from the anterior pituitary. Conventionally, the ability of the pituitary to release PRL in vivo is usually tested by administration of drugs blocking dopamine action at the postsynaptic receptor (haloperidol, metochlopramide, chlorpromazine) by TRH, and finally by insulin-induced hypoglycemia. Less frequently, sleep studies are used for such a purpose. The suppressibility of the system is tested by measuring serum PRL after the administration of a single dose of apomorphine or bromoncriptine (Tolis and Francs, 1979).

According to most investigators basal serum PRL levels seem to be normal in depressed patients. Similarly, the lactotrope suppressibility does not differ between control subjects and depressed patients. In a recent study of patients with major endogenous depressed disorders, it was reported that there was a statistically significant elevation of PRL during the evening, several hours before sleep (Hallbreich and co-workers, 1979). In contrast, there was no difference at any other time, and the nocturnal PRL output was similar to that of control subjects. Whether this difference was due to a stress factor was not evaluated, since no concomittant ACTH rhythms were performed. Nevertheless, in spite of its limitations, the study did confirm that the evaluation of PRL in the evening correlated with alterations in mood. The study should be repeated in a more homogenous population with the same type of depressive disorder, and the data should be compared to a suitable group matched for age. It may also prove fruitful to compare either catecholamine and serotonin metabolites in such circadian studies, and/or platelet monoamine oxidase activity, the latter of which seems to correlate with plasm PRL under specific pharmacological situations (Kleinman and co-workers, 1979).

Provocative tests for PRL secretion have used mainly TRH as a secretagogue. From limited studies it appears that in contrast to patients with mania, patients with depressive states show a reduced PRL output (Meada and co-workers, 1975; Mendlewicz and co-workers, 1980). This seems to be true primarily for postmenopausal women in particular (Mendlewicz and co-workers, 1980). Whether estrogen ameliorates the state of the depression or the PRL responses has not yet been explored.

Miscellaneous

Melatonin

Recent studies have shown that in depression there is an abnormal 24 hour pattern of melatonin levels-there is no nocturnal increase as found in normal subjects (Mendlewicz and co-workers, 1979b). The interpretation of this finding is problematical, since the quality of sleep was not reported in the study. The finding may, however, point to a disturbance of the pineal hypothalamic circuit. Recently a similar abnormality was observed in patients with anorexia nervosa (Brown, 1981). Whether specific neuropharmacological agents can restore the normal rhythm is as yet unknown. Finally, whether persistence of the abnormality in "treated patients" will herald a potential relapse has yet to be determined.

Calcitonin

Calcitonin-receptors have been identified in various hypothalamic and extra hypothalamic areas, but their significance remains a mystery. Recently, it was reported that administration of calcitonin, resulting in a decreased serum calcium and increased CSF calcium, led to diminished arousal and enhanced depressive scores (Carman and Wyatt, 1979). Since a decrease in CSF calcium has been reported during improvement of the depressive illness, it may be rewarding to examine furher the role of calciotropic hormones (Vitamin D, parathormone, and calcitonin) in subjects with manic-depressive illnesses. To what extent such agents have therapeutic applications remains to be determined.

Opioid Peptides (encephalins, endorphins, b-lipotropin)

Beta lipotropin is a pituitary hormone of still debatable physiological significance. "Fragments" of it are capable of inducing specific behavioral effects and analgesia. Their presence has been demonstrated in a group of psychotic patients who underwent dialysis (Palmour, 1977) and their involvement in the pathophysiology of mental illness has been presumed on the basis of data showing that blockade of their receptor sites by naloxone results in improvement insome catatonics (Gunne and co-workers, 1977). Measurements of the levels of any of the opioid peptides in blood, CSF, or other biological fluids have not been reported with regard to manic-depressive illnesses. On the other hand, studies employing endorphin-related hormonal release have been reported but are as yet preliminary (Catlin and co-workers, 1980). In view of the fact that opioid peptides may, like antipsychotic medications, enhance pituitary PRL release, it is theoretically possible to correlate anti-schizophrenic actions of classical drugs and PRL release.

Systematic long- term studies using refined technology are needed in order to collect precise rather than anecdotal data that will lead to a better understanding of the biology of depressive disorders. These studies should evaluate both the metabolic fate of the classical neurotransmitters and the functional status of the hypothalamic-pituitary axis. Studies of postmortem material, evaluation of monoamine metabolism, determination of concentrations of neurotransmitters in blood and tissues (CNS), neuropeptides, and hormones, pharmacological manipulation of central "neurotransmitter" tone, and finally detailed neuroendocrine testing may provide psychobiologists with "a window on the brain of patients with depressive illness" (De la Fuente and Rosenbaum, 1979).

REFERENCES

Altman, N., E.J. Sachar, P.H. Gruen, F.S. Halpern, and E.Eto (1975). Psychosom. Med., 37, 274-276.
Amsterdam, J.D., A. Winokur, J. Mendels, and P. Snyder (1979). Lancet, 2, 904-905.
Asnis, G.M., P.S. Nathan, U. Halbreich, F.S. Halpern, and E.J. Sachar (1980). Lancet, 1, 425.
Brown, G.M., J.A. Seggie, and J.W. Chambers (1978). Psychoneuroendocrinology, 3, 131-154.
Brown, W.A., R. Johnston, and D. Mayfield (1979). Am. J. Psychiat., 136, 543-547.
Brown, G. (1981). Personal communication.
Carman, J.S., and R.J. Wyatt (1979). Arch. Gen. Psychiat., 36, 72-75.
Carroll, B.J. (1969). Br. Med. J., 3, 27-28.
Carroll, B.J., and J. Mendels (1976a). In E. Sachar (Ed.), Hormones, Behavior and Psychopathology, Raven Press, New York. pp. 193-224.
Carroll, B.J., and J. Mendels (1976b). Arch. Gen. Psychiat., 33, 1051-1058.
Catlin, D.H., R.E. Poland, D.A. Corelick, R.H. Gerner, K.K. Hui, R.T. Rubin, and C.H. Li (1980). J. Clin. Endocrinol. Metab., 50, 1021.
Chazot, G. (1974). Lyon Med., 231, 831-836.
De la Fuente, J.R., and A.H. Rosenbaum (1979). Mayo Clin. Proc., 54, 109-118.
DeLeon-Jones, F., J.W. Maas, H. Dekirmenjian, and J. Sanchez (1975). Am. J. Psychiat., 132, 1141-1148.
Ehrensing, R.H., A.J. Kastin, D.S. Schalch, H.G.Friesen, J.R. Vargas, and A.V. Schally (1974). Am. J. Psychiat., 131, 714-718.
Endo, M., J. Endo, M. Nishikubo, T. Yamaguchi, and N. Hatotani (1974). In N. Hatotani (Ed.), Psychoneuroendocrinology, Karger, Basel. pp. 22-31.
Extein, I., A.L.C. Rottash, and M.S. Gold (1980). N. Engl. J. Med., 302, 923-924.
Fisher, R.C. Schiavi, A. Edwards, D.M. Davis, M. Reitman, and J. Fine (1979). Arch. Gen. Psychiat., 36, 431-437.
Gessa, G.L., E. Paglietti, and B.P. Cuarantotti (1980). Science, 203-205.
Gold, E.M. (1980). In D.T. Krieger, and J.C. Hughes (Eds.), Neuroendocrinology, Sinauer Press, New York. pp.311-320.
Gold, P., E.De Fraites, and A.P. Zis (1980). Psychopharmacol. Bull., 16, 36-38.
Gruen, P.H., E.J. Sachar, N. Altman, and J. Sassin (1975). Arch. Gen. Psychiat., 32, 31-33.
Gunne, M.L., L. Lindstrom, and L. Terenius (1977). J. Neurol. Trans., 40, 13-19.
Halbreich, U., L. Grunhaus, and M. Ben-David (1979). Arch. Gen. Psychiat., 36, 1183-1186.
Hollister, L.E., P. Berger, F.L. Ongle, R.C. Arnold, and A. Johnson (1975). Psychopharmacol. Bull., 11, 27-28.
Karlberg, B.E., B.F. Kjelman. and B. Kagedal (1978). Acta Psychiat. Scand., 58, 389-400.
Kirkegaard, C., and N. Bjorum (1980). Lancet, 1, 152.
Kleinman, J.E., A. Rogol, M.S. Buchsbaum, D.L. Murphy, J.C. Gillin, H.A. Nasrallah, and R.J. Wyatt (1979). Science, 206, 479-481.
Loosen, P.T., and A.J. Prange (1980). N. Engl. J. Med., 303, 224-225.
Maeda, K., Y. Kato, S. Ohgo, K. Chihara, Y. Yoshimoto, N. Yamaguchi, S. Kuromaru, and H. Imura (1975). J. Clin. Endocrinol. Metab., 40, 501-505.
Martin, J.B. (1979). In G. Tolis (Ed.), Clinical Neuroendocrinology: a pathophysiologic approach, Raven Press, New York. pp. 269-278.
Matussek N. (1977). In Depressive Disorders, Hoechst Medical Symposium No. 13, Schattauer Verlag, Stuttgart. pp. 431-436.
Mendlewicz, J., P. Linkowski, and H. Brauman (1979a). Lancet, 2, 1079.
Mendlewicz, J., P. Linkowski, L. Branchey, U. Weinberg, E.D. Weitzman, and M. Branchey (1979b). Lancet, 2, 1362.
Mendlewicz, J., P. Linkowski, and H. Brauman (1980). N. Engl. J. Med., 302, 1091-1092.
Moss, R.L., and S.M. Mc Cann (1975). Science, 181, 177-179.

Mueller, P.S., G.R. Heninger, and R.K. Mc Donald (1969). Arch. Gen. Psychiat., 21, 587-594.
Naftolin, F., and G. Tolis (1978). Clin. Obst. Gyn., 21, 17-29.
Ojeida, S.R., and S.M. Mc Cann (1974). Neuroendocrinology, 12, 295-315.
Palmour, R. (1977). Abstracts of the Society of Neuroscience. pp. 32.
Perez-Reys, M. (1972). In T. Williams (Ed.), Recent Advances in the Psychobiology of the Depressive Illnesses, Government Printing Office, Washington D.C. pp. 131-135.
Prange, A.J., and I.C. Wilson (1972). Psychopharmacologia (Berlin), Suppl. 26, 82.
Renaud, L.P., H.W. Blume, O.J. Pittman, Y. Lamour, and A.T. Tan (1979). Science, 205, 1275-1277.
Sachar, E.J., J. Finkelstein, and L. Hellman (1971). Arch. Gen. Psychiat., 25, 263-269.
Sachar, E.J. (1973). In J. Mendels (Ed.), Biological Psychiatry, J. Wiley, New York. pp. 175-197.
Sachar, E.J. (1974). Am. J. Psychiat., 131, 608-609.
Schlesser, M.A., G. Winokur, and B.M. Sherman (1979). Lancet, 1, 739-741.
Snyder, F. (1968). In N.S. Kline and E. Laska (Eds.), Computers and Electronic Devices in Psychiatry, Grune-Stratton, New York. pp. 272-303.
Takahashi, S., H. Kondo, and M. Yoshimura (1973). Folia Psychiat. Neurol. Jap., 27, 305-314.
Tolis, G., G. Bertrand, and E. Pilter (1973). Psychosom. Med., 41, 657-659.
Tolis, G., R. Dent, and H. Guyda (1978). J. Clin. Endocrinol. Metab., 47, 200-203.
Tolis, G., and S.Francs (1979). In G. Tolis, F. Labrie, J. Martin, and F. Naftolin (Eds.), Clinical Neuroendocrinology: A Pathophysiologic Approach, Raven Press, New York. pp. 291-318.
Tolis, G., L. Jukier, H. Guyda, and D. Krieger (1979a). Clin. Res., 27, 261.
Tolis, G., J.M. McKenzie, J.B. Martin, and G. Bertrand (1979b). In G. Tolis, F. Labrie, J. Martin, and F. Naftolin (Eds.), Clinical Neuroendocrinology: A Pathophysiologic Approach, Raven Press, New York. pp. 437-448.
Tolis, G. (1980). In D. Krieger, and J. Hughes (Eds.), Neuroendocrinology, Sinauer Press, New York. pp. 321-330.
Tolis, G., D. Goltzman, and H. Gnyda (1980). J. Endocrinol. Invest., 3, 83-97.
Tolis, G. (1981). Psychosom. Med. (In Press)
Vagenakis, A. (1979). In G. Tolis, F. Labrie, J. Martin, and F. Naftolin (Eds.), Clinical Neuroendocrinology: A Pathophysiologic Arproach, Raven Press, New York. pp. 329-343.
Weisenburger, D.D., G.L. Fry, and J.C. Hoak (1980). Lancet, 1, 100.
Yen, S.S.C. (1980). In D. Krieger, and J.C. Hughes (Eds.), Neuroendocrinology, Sinauer Press, New York. pp. 255-274.

Thyrotropin and Prolactin Responses to Thyrotropin-Releasing Hormone Stimulation Test in Male Inpatients with Psychotic and Neurotic Depression

A. Martinos[*], D. N. Papachristou[**], P. Rinieris[*], A. Souvatzoglou[**], D. A. Koutras[**] and C. Stefanis[*]

[*]Department of Psychiatry, University of Athens, Eginition Hospital, Athens, Greece
[**]Department of Clinical Therapeutics, University of Athens, Alexandra's Hospital, Athens, Greece

ABSTRACT

We investigated the thyrotropin (TSH) and prolactin (PRL) responses to thyrotropin-releasing hormone (TRH) stimulation test, performed at 14.00 and 24.00 hours, in 19 male psychotic depressives, 11 male neurotic depressives and 10 mentally healthy men.
No significant differences were detected between the groups of psychotic depressives, neurotic depressives and normal controls with regard to TSH_0, TSH_{30}, ΔTSH, PRL_0, PRL_{30} and ΔPRL values at 14.00 and 24.00 hours. However, only in the group of psychotic depressives the mean TSH_0, TSH_{30} and ΔTSH values at 24.00 hours were found significantly higher than those at 14.00 hours

KEYWORDS

Thyrotropin-releasing hormone stimulation test; prolactin; thyrotropin; psychotic depression; neurotic depression.

INTRODUCTION

Thyrotropin-releasing hormone (TRH) stimulates thyrotropin (TSH) and prolactin (PRL) release in normal subjects (Maeda and co-workers, 1975). In psychotic depressives the TSH responses to TRH stimulation test have varied from normal to decreased (Kastin and co-workers, 1972; Prange and co-workers, 1972; Coppen and co-workers, 1974; Ehrensing and co-workers, 1974; Kirkgaard and co-workers, 1975; Maeda and co-workers, 1975; Hollister and co-workers, 1976; Gold and co-workers, 1977; Linnoila and co-workers, 1979). Abnormal PRL responses to TRH stimulation have been found in psychotic depressives (Ehrensing and co-workers, 1974; Maeda and co-workers, 1975; Linnoila and co-workers, 1979). However, the results in three studies concerning the PRL response are contradictory. In one of them exaggerated (Maeda and co-workers, 1975) and in the other two blunted responses were observed in the minority (Ehrensing and co-workers, 1974) or the majority of the patients (Linnoila and co-workers, 1979).
The TRH stimulation test-performed in the morning-in patients with psychotic or neurotic depression showed decreased TSH responses in the psychotic depressives compared to those found in the neurotic depressives and the controls (Kirkgaard

and co-workers, 1978).
Since there is a circadian variation of plasma TSH in normal subjects with lower levels in the day-time and higher levels at night, and the TSH level is rather constant between 11.00 and 20.00 hours and between 23.00 and 8.00 hours, TSH measurement on one blood sample obtained from each of the above-mentioned two intervals would be sufficient to estimate the magnitude of the circadian variation of TSH (Weeke and Weeke, 1978). Thus, Weeke and Weeke (1978) investigated the circadian variation of serum TSH - by obtaining two blood samples from each patient at 14.00 and 24.00 hours - in a group of psychotic depressives and found a diminution or absence of the night increase of TSH in severely depressed patients.
The above findings prompted us to investigate the TSH and PRL responses to TRH stimulation test performed at 14.00 and 24.00 hours in male inpatients with psychotic depression and neurotic depression. It must be noted that the group of psychotic depressives was unselected with regard to depression's diagnostic subtype (i.e. unipolar, bipolar or involutional depression).

METHOD

Material in the present study consisted of 30 male depressed patients, hospitalized at Eginition Hospital (Department of Psychiatry, University of Athens). Patients were assigned to the study group solely on the basis of the following criteria: 1) abstinence from psychotropic drugs for at least three weeks prior to admission, and 2) absence of overt clinical symptoms or of history indicating thyroid or other endocrinological disease.
Nineteen of our patients were diagnosed as psychotic and 11 as neurotic depressives. The diagnosis was made by two independent assessors (P.R. and A.M.) according to the diagnostic criteria of Sinanan and co-workers (1975). The age of the patients ranged from 24 to 62 years with a mean of 55.3 ± 7.4 for the psychotic depressives and of 45.1 ± 8.6 for the neurotics. There was a significant difference between the mean ages of the two groups ($p<0.01$).
The group of psychotic depressives consisted of 4 patients with bipolar depression, 3 with unipolar depression and 12 with involutional depression. Kupfer and co-workers' (1975) modification of the diagnostic criteria of Perris (1966) was used for the diagnosis of bipolar and unipolar depression. Thus, to be considered as suffering from bipolar depression, patients were required to have had at least one documented episode of hypomania or mania and at least one episode of clinical depression, while to be considered as suffering from unipolar depression, it was required that the reason for seeking psychiatric care was for the treatment of depression, that the past history was negative for hypomania and mania, and that the patients had had at least two previous episodes of depression severe enough to warrant antidepressant medication (Kupfer and co-workers, 1975). The diagnosis of involutional depression was made according to the American Psychiatric Association's (DSM-II, 1968) description of involutional melancholia. Thus, to be considered as suffering from involutional depression, it was required that the reason for seeking psychiatric care was for the treatment of severe depression starting within the involutional phase of life (age of 50-65 years for men - Rosenthal, 1968) and characterized by worry, anxiety, agitation, severe insomnia, feelings of guilt and somatic pre occupations, and that the past history was negative for mental disorder.
All patients were placed under the same nursing care and diet. Following admission each patient was allowed 1 week's period of adaptation in the ward, during which he received 10mg of diazepam every evening. On the day of TRH testing, i.e. following the week's adaptation period, diazepam was discontinued and the mental state of the patients was reassessed by one of the authors (A.M.) with the aid of Hamilton's (1960) rating scale for depression (HDRS). The TRH stimulation test was performed at 14.00 and 24.00 hours. Blood samples were drawn from an antecubital

Thyrotropin and Prolactin Responses

vein before and 30 min after the intravenous injection of 200 μg TRH for determination of TSH and PRL. The sera were stored at $-20°C$ until analyzed. The pituitary hormones were measured by radioimmunoassays.
The results obtained in the two groups of patients were compared to a control group consisting of 10 mentally healthy men, aged 26 to 65 years (mean 48.5 years), who were found without somatic diseases known to influence the TSH and PRL responses to TRH.
Hormonal determinations were carried out at the Endocrine Laboratory of the Department of Clinical Therapeutics of Athens University (Alexandra Hospital).
For the statistical analyses the Wilcoxon test was used and Spearman's rank-order correlation coefficients were computed.

RESULTS

The mean basal TSH level (TSH_0), the mean TSH level 30 min after the TRH injection (TSH_{30}) and the mean ΔTSH (i.e. the difference between TSH_0 and TSH_{30} values) at 24.00 hours were higher (but not to statistically significant degrees) than those at 14.00 hours in the groups of neurotic depressives and normal controls.
In the group of psychotic depressives the mean TSH_0, TSH_{30} and ΔTSH values at 24.00 hours were significantly higher than those at 14.00 hours ($p<0.01$, $p<0.01$ and $p<0.05$ respectively) (Table 1).

TABLE 1. Serum TSH, μU/ml (Mean ± SE), in psychotic depressives

Time	TSH_0	TSH_{30}	ΔTSH
14.00	0.8±0.1	9.2±1.0	8.4±0.9
24.00	1.6±0.3*	12.0±1.3*	10.4±1.1**

*$p<0.01$ **$p<0.05$

The mean basal PRL level (PRL_0) at 24.00 hours was higher (but not to a statistically significant degree) than that at 14.00 hours in all the investigated groups. The mean PRL level 30 min after the TRH injection (PRL_{30}) at 24.00 hours was significantly lower than that at 14.00 hours in all our groups ($p<0.05$) (Table 2).

TABLE 2. PRL_{30}, ng/ml (Mean ± SE), in our material

Subjects	14.00	24.00
Psychotic depressives (N=19)	78.1±11.5	57.9±7.6*
Neurotic depressives (N=11)	74.3± 8.1	57.7±7.0*
Normal controls (N=10)	64.2± 8.2	48.3±8.3*

*$p<0.05$

The mean ΔPRL (i.e. the difference between PRL_0 and PRL_{30} values) at 24.00 hours was lower (but not to a statistically significant degree) than that at 14.00 hours in all the groups.
No significant difference was found between the groups of psychotic depressives, neurotic depressives and normal controls with regard to TSH_0, TSH_{30}, ΔTSH, PRL_0, PRL_{30} and ΔPRL values at 14.00 and 24.00 hours (Wilcoxon test for unpaired measurements).
There was no significant correlation of the HDRS total score (or the score of any of this scale's behavioral items) with the values of TSH_0, TSH_{30}, ΔTSH, PRL_0,

PRL_{30} and ΔPRL in the groups of psychotic and neurotic depressives.

DISCUSSION

In our study no significant differences were detected between the groups of psychotic depressives, neurotic depressives and normal controls with regard to TSH_0, TSH_{30}, ΔTSH, PRL_0, PRL_{30} and ΔPRL values at 14.00 and 24.00 hours.
Since only in the group of psychotic depressives the mean TSH_0, TSH_{30} and TSH values at 24.00 hours were found significantly higher than those at 14.00 hours, this finding might be specifically related to this psychopathological condition. It has been reported that TSH response to TRH stimulation test is decreased in unipolar depressed patients (Prange and co-workers, 1972; Gold and co-workers, 1977). The fact that we did not observe a reduced TSH response in our sample of psychotic depressives might be attributed to the presence of only 3 unipolar depressed patients in this sample. More over the absence of a decreased TSH response in our involutional depressed patients who prevailed in our sample, might suggest that unipolar and involutional depressed patients differ in their response to TRH test. Further research, however, is needed to confirm the validity of these results and their clinical usefulness.

REFERENCES

Coppen, A., S. Montgomery, M. Peet, J. Bailey, V. Marks, and P. Woods (1974). Lancet, 2, 433-435.
Ehrensing, R.H., A.J. Kastin, D.S. Schalch, H.G. Friesen, J.R. Vargas, and A.V. Schally (1974). Am. J. Psychiat., 131, 714-718.
Gold, P.W., F.K. Goodwin, T. Wehr, and R. Rebar (1977). Am. J. Psychiat., 134, 1028-1031.
Hamilton, M. (1960). J.Neurol. Neurosurg. Psychiat., 23, 53-62.
Hollister, L.E., K.L. Davis, and P.A. Berger (1976). Arch. Gen. Psychiat., 33, 1393-1396.
Kastin, A.J., R.H. Ehrensing, D.S. Schalch, and M.S. Anderson (1972). Lancet, 2, 740-742.
Kirkegaard, C., N. Norlem, U.B. Lauridsen, N. Bjorum, and C. Christiansen (1975). Arch. Gen. Psychiat., 32, 1115-1118.
Kirkegaard, C., N. Bjorum, D. Cohn, and U.B.Lauridsen (1978). Arch. Gen. Psychiat. 35, 1017-1021.
Kupfer, D.J., D. Pickar, J.M. Himmelhoch, and T.P. Detre (1975). Arch. Gen. Psychiat., 32, 866-871.
Linnoila, M., B.A. Lamberg, G. Rosberg, S.L. Karonen, and M.G. Welin (1979). Acta Psychiat. Scand., 59, 536-544.
Maeda, K., Y.Kato, S. Ohgo, K. Chihara, Y. Yoshimoto, N. Yamaguchi, S. Kuromaru, and H. Imura (1975). J. Clin. Endocrinol. Metab., 40, 501-505.
Perris, C. (1966). Acta Psychiat. Scand., Suppl. 194.
Prange, A.J., I.C. Wilson, P.P. Lara, L.B. Alltop, and G.R. Breese (1972). Lancet, 2, 999-1002.
Rosenthal, S.H. (1968). Am. J. Psychiat., 124, 21-35.
Sinanan, K., A.M.B. Keatinge, P.G.S. Beckett, and W.C. Love (1975). Br. J. Psychiat., 126, 49-55.
Weeke, A., and J. Weeke (1978). Acta Psychiat. Scand., 57, 281-289.

5. Treatment Aspects of Depression

Current Treatment for Depression

P. Kielholz

University Psychiatric Clinic, Basle, Switzerland

ABSTRACT

1. According to the results of all recent epidemiological enquiries, the number of cases of depression diagnosed is increasing. Parallel with this, a clear trend towards a change in the symptomatology in the direction of masked depression has been observed.
2. 80-90% of all cases of depression are now being diagnosed and treated by general practitioners. Ambulant treatment by doctors who are not themselves psychiatrists is thus assuming ever-greater importance. It was for this reason that an International Committee for Prevention and Treatment of Depression has been founded by us with the aim of educating general practitioners in the diagnosis and treatment of depression and improving collaboration between general practitioners and psychiatrists.
3. Essential for the success of treatment is a carefully established diagnosis, in which the nosological classification determines the indication for basic treatment and the phenomenological diagnosis the indication for the choice of the right antidepressant.
4. Depressive patients should be informed in advance about the delayed onset of action of antidepressants, as well as about their potential side effects.
5. Therapy-resistant endogenous depressions can frequently be overcome by resorting to intravenous drip infusions, i.e. infusions containing nomifensine (Alival) for cases of retarded depression, and a combination of clomipramine (Anafranil) and maprotiline (Ludiomil)in cases of depression with strong overtones of anxiety. Such intravenous therapy has been observed to speed up the onset of the mood-brightening effect of these antidepressants.

KEY WORDS

Masked depression; depressive states; nosological classification; somatic depressions; basic treatment; antidepressants; psychotherapy.

INTRODUCTION

According to the results of all recent epidemiological enquiries, depressions are currently on the increase in all the so-called civilised countries, especially in urban surroundings (Berner et al. 1973, Fazio 1973, Hakim 1973, Helmchen 1973, Kielholz 1973). This apparent increase is largely to be attributed to an improvement in the diagnosis of depressive states. Parallel with this, it is possible to detect a clear trend towards a change in the symptomatology of depression in the direction of somatisation, i.e. in the direction of masked depression. These masked depressions are often diagnosed too late or even not at all. We should therefore centre our graduate and post-graduate education even more on the recognition and diagnosis of masked depressions.

We apply the term masked depression to endogenous or psychogenic depressive illnesses in which the somatic symptoms occupy the foreground, or in which the psychic symptoms recede into the background. Masked depression is thus a phenomenological diagnosis.

Presented schematically in Figure 1 is the current concept of masked depressions.

FIGURE 1. Masked depression (cardinal features of the syndrome)

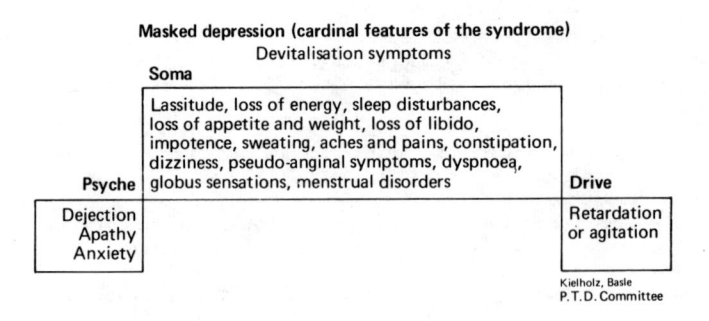

Masked depression (cardinal features of the syndrome)
Devitalisation symptoms

Psyche	Soma	Drive
Dejection Apathy Anxiety	Lassitude, loss of energy, sleep disturbances, loss of appetite and weight, loss of libido, impotence, sweating, aches and pains, constipation, dizziness, pseudo-anginal symptoms, dyspnoea, globus sensations, menstrual disorders	Retardation or agitation

Kielholz, Basle
P.T.D. Committee

One should only make a diagnosis of masked depression in cases where the presence of a depressive state can definitely be established. The physical mask of the depression may consist in a wide variety of autonomic nervous disturbances and organ-related symptoms of functional origin and are therefore liable to mimic the symptomatology of almost any illness. The variety and frequency of the autonomic nervous symptoms are indicated in Figure 2.

FIGURE 2. Autonomic nervous disturbances and organ-related symptoms of functional origin

Masked depression

Autonomic nervous disturbances and organ-related symptoms of functional origin accompanied by unobtrusive depressive manifestations.

In all patients presenting with somatic disorders it is of course necessary to carry out a thorough physical examination. Provided a carefully recorded case history and a thorough physical examination disclose no evidence of a somatic illness, a more detailed examination of the case history and specific questioning of the patient should be undertaken with a view to lifting the mask of physical symptoms and uncovering the depressive syndrome concealed behind it (Kielholz et al 1978). The following list of questions drawn up by the WHO has proved most useful in helping to expose a depressive symptomatology lurking in the background.

FIGURE 3. Examples of key-questions

Concrete questions which the patient should be asked

1. Do you still get any enjoyment out of life?
2. Do you find it difficult to make decisions?
3. Are there certain things that still interest you?
4. Have you lately been tending to brood more than usual?
5. Do you have the feeling that life for you has become pointless?
6. Do you feel tired and devoid of energy?
7. Do you have any trouble with your sleep?
8. Do you feel pain anywhere, or perhaps a sensation of pressure in the chest?
9. Do you have a poor appetite, or have you been losing weight?
10. Have you any difficulties of a sexual kind?

Particular attention should be devoted to the following symptoms, which can be regarded as strengthening one's suspicions of a depression: loss of the ability to experience pleasure, difficulty in making decisions, loss of interest, a tendency to brooding, and a shift in basic mood towards the direction of sadness, anxiety, or apathy (Dilling et al 1978, Kielholz et al 1979).
The greater the number of depressive signs found to be present during a direct exploration, the greater the likelihood that the patient is in a depressive state. If an exact case history - which of course should also cover the patient's heredity, the course of his illness, and his familial, professional, and psychosocial environmental situation - lends further support to one's suspicions of a depressive illness, the next step is to make a dual recording in the form of a nosological and phenomenological diagnosis.

FIGURE 4. Nosological classification

Nosological classification of depressive states

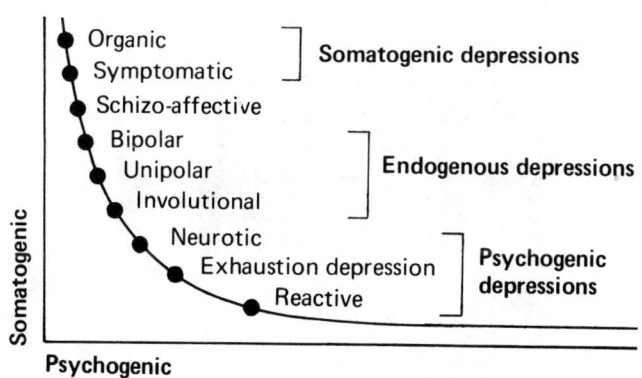

- Organic
- Symptomatic   } Somatogenic depressions
- Schizo-affective
- Bipolar
- Unipolar   } Endogenous depressions
- Involutional
- Neurotic
- Exhaustion depression } Psychogenic depressions
- Reactive

(y-axis: Somatogenic; x-axis: Psychogenic)

This nosological classification has proved very useful, because from it the basic therapy, the clinical course, and the prognosis can be directly inferred. It has also been taken over by the WHO in its 9th Revision of the International Classification of Diseases, which came into force on 1st January 1980.

Every depressive patient should first be subjected to a thorough physical and neurological examination, in order to ensure that cases of somatogenic depression - to which the pharmacogenic depressions also belong - are recognised. A somatogenic depression may be of the organic type, i.e. due to morphological changes in the brain, or it may be of the symptomatic type. Depressions may sometimes be preceded by organic diseases, e.g. by cancer, heart failure, or incipient cerebral arteriosclerosis; they may also occur during convalescence after infectious diseases or after drug or alcohol abuse, e.g. in patients recovering from hepatitis or influenza or in those who have been dependent on psychomotor amines. It is important to take a case history of drug consumption, in order to preclude the possibility of a pharmacogenic depression.

FIGURE 5. Somatic depressions

Somatogenic depressions	Pathogenesis	Therapy
Organic	Morphological changes in the brain, as for example in cerebral arteriosclerosis, senile dementia, craniocerebral injuries, brain tumours, progressive paralysis, epilepsy, oligophrenia	Treatment for the underlying disease possibly together with prescription of an antidepressant
Symptomatic	Infectious diseases, e.g. hepatitis, influenza, pneumonia Cardiovascular disorders Endocrine diseases Withdrawal of alcohol or drugs in addicts	Therapy depending on the nature of the causative factors possibly together with prescription of an antidepressant
Pharmacogenic	Reserpine-containing antihypertensives Major tranquillisers Corticosteroids Oral contraceptives	Withdrawal of the medication

Of course, in cases of somatogenic depression, the underlying somatic disease has to be treated first. In a patient with arteriosclerotic depression, for example, it is often possible to eliminate the depression promptly simply by prescribing treatment for his incipient heart failure.

As I have already mentioned, the indication for basic therapy can be inferred from the nosological diagnosis.

FIGURE 6. Basic treatment for depressions

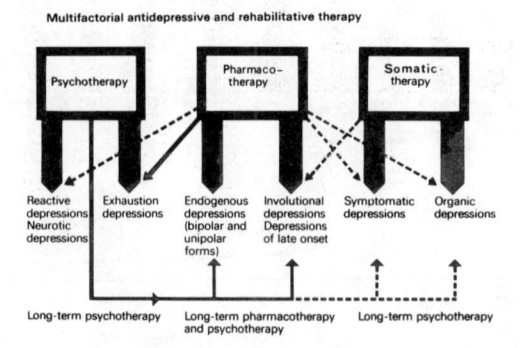

As it can be seem from Figure 6, a combination of psychotherapy and pharmacotherapy is necessary both in psychogenic and in endogenous depressions. Unfortunately, a nosological diagnosis is not sufficient in itself to ensure the success of treatment; the phenomenological aspects must be considered too. Here, a distinction has to be made between four main target symptoms (as defined by Freyhan 1960, 1961): sadness and dejection, anxiety and agitation, retardation and apathy, or psychosomatic masking symptoms.

FIGURE 7. Phenomenological diagnosis

> Clinical picture of the depression predominantly characterised by:
> 1. Sadness, dejection, despondency
> 2. Anxiety, apprehensiveness, anxious agitation
> 3. Retardation, sluggishness, lack of drive, apathy
> 4. Physical symptoms, autonomic nervous dysfunction, and functional disturbances referable to specific organs or organ systems (masked depression)
>
> Kielholz, Basle
> P.T.D. Committee

Essential for the success of treatment is selection of the right antidepressant for the right patient in the right dosage. The antidepressants available today exhibit three principal properties to varying degrees, i.e. an effect which is either primarily mood-brightening, primarily anxiolytic, or primarily drive-enhancing (Angst 1961, 1963).
By reference to their activity profiles the antidepressants can be divided into three main groups:

FIGURE 8. Activity profiles of antidepressants

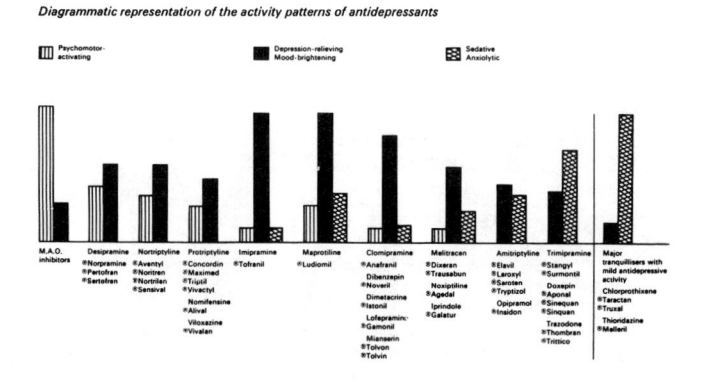

FIGURE 9. Antidepressants with differing activity profiles

Antidepressants with differing activity profiles

M.A.O. inhibitors	Desipramine	Imipramine	Maprotiline	Amitriptyline	Thioridazine
JATROSOM	NORPRAMINE	TOFRANIL	LUDIOMIL	ELAVIL	MELLERIL
MARPLAN	PERTOFRAN			LAROXYL	
NIAMID	SERTOFREN	Clomipramine		SAROTEN	Flupentixol
		ANAFRANIL		TRYPTIZOL	FLUANXOL
	Nortriptyline				
	AVENTYL	Dibenzepin		Trimipramine	Chlorprothixene
	NORITREN	NOVERIL		STANGYL	TARACTAN
	NOTRILEN			SURMONTIL	TRUXAL
	SENSIVAL	Melitracen			
		DIXERAN		Doxepin	Levomepromazine
	Protriptyline	TRAUSABUN		APONAL	NEUROCIL
	CONCORDIN			SINEQUAN	NOZINAN
	TRIPTIL	Dimetracine		SINQUAN	VERACTIL
	VIVACTYL	ISTONIL			
					Opipramol
	Nomifensine	Noxiptiline			INSIDON
	ALIVAL	AGEDAL			
		Iprindole			
		GALATUR			
		Mianserin			
		TOLVON			

By reference to these activity profiles it is possible to determine relatively easily which type of antidepressant is indicated in a given case. One should in fact prescribe whichever antidepressant has an activity profile most suited to the phenomenological diagnosis.
If the predominant phenomenological symptoms of the depression are inhibition of thought processes, apathy, and lack of drive, an antidepressant with a drive-enhancing and activating effect should be prescribed, e.g. nomifensine (Alival). On the other hand, if the clinical picture is mainly characterised by anxiety, mental unrest, or anxious agitation, an antidepressant with a primarily anxiolytic effect is indicated, e.g. amitriptyline (Laroxyl, Saroten) or trimipramine (Surmontil).
Unfortunately, all antidepressants known to date have a delayed onset of action and are apt to provoke various side effects at the beginning of treatment. In our opinion, it is therefore advisable to draw the patient's attention in advance to the fact that the medication will have a delayed onset of action and that side effects may occur at the start of treatment.

These side effects are partly due to the anticholinergic properties of the antidepressants. Side effects such as dryness of the mouth, sweating, blurring of vision, and occasionally also tachycardia may prove particularly unpleasant for the patient during the initial stage of treatment.
The drive-enhancing antidepressants usually have less marked side effects than antidepressants with an anxiolytic action. If one omits to tell the patients in advance about the delayed onset of action of antidepressants, as well as about their side effects, they lose confidence both in the drug and in the physician when side effects appear: and, especially if they are being treated on an ambulant basis, they are then liable simply to stop taking the drug.

FIGURE 10. Side effects of antidepressants

Accompanying effects of treatment with antidepressants

Type of effect	Incidence		
	M.A.O. inhibitors	Antidepressants mood-brightening	
		drive-enhancing	anxiety-relieving
Autonomic nervous symptoms:			
Dryness of the mouth	–	•	•••
Sweating	(*)	•	•••
Blurring of vision	–	•	•••
Constipation	•	•	••
Dizziness	•••	•	••
Postural hypotension	•••	(*)	••
Disturbances of micturition, retention of urine	–	•	•
Tachycardia	••	•	•
E.C.G. changes	(*)	(*)	(*)
Hypertensive crises	•	–	–
Extrapyramidal symptoms:			
Fine tremor of the fingers	–	(*)	•
General condition:			
Tiredness, somnolence	–	–	•
Inner restlessness	••	••	(*)
Sleep disturbances	••	••	–
Psychopathological symptoms:			
Activation of schizophrenic symptoms	••	••	(*)
Sudden change from depressive to manic phase	•	••	•
Deliria	–	•	••
Increase in cerebral excitability	–	(*)	(*)

Psychotherapy

As already seen on Figure 6 dealing with basic treatment for depressions, the greater the extent to which psychogenic elements predominate in the origin of a depression, the greater the extent to which psychotherapy is indicated. Any form of antidepressive pharmacotherapy is bound to fail unless it is also accompanied by psychotherapy. In no other type of psychic disorder are so many errors committed as in the treatment of depression. It is the similarity which depression bears to physiological sadness which is largely responsible for these therapeutic errors. We have thersfore tried to pinpoint in Figure 11 the commonest errors made in the psychotherapeutic approach to depressive patients.

FIGURE 11. What one should NOT do

WHAT ONE SHOULD NOT DO:

1. URGE THE PATIENT TO PULL HIMSELF TOGETHER
2. SEND HIM ON HOLIDAY OR TO A SPA
3. ALLOW HIM TO TAKE IMPORTANT DECISIONS
4. CAST DOUBT ON HIS DELUSIONAL IDEAS
5. ASSERT THAT HIS CONDITION IS ALREADY IMPROVING

It is also essential to ensure that the depressive patient is precisely informed about his illness and its treatment.

FIGURE 12. What one SHOULD bo

WHAT ONE SHOULD DO:

1. ACCEPT THE PATIENT AND HIS ILLNESS
2. EMPHASISE THAT THE ILLNESS HAS A FAVOURABLE PROGNOSIS
3. EXPLAIN THE PLAN OF TREATMENT TO THE PATIENT
4. DRAW HIS ATTENTION TO THE SIDE EFFECTS OF THE MEDICATION
5. MENTION THAT THE PATIENT MAY EXPERIENCE TRANSIENT MOOD FLUCTUATIONS
6. SET SHORT-TERM THERAPEUTIC AIMS FOR THE PATIENT, SO THAT HE CAN EXPERIENCE SUCCESSES

Another important point is to reassure the patient again and again that his depression can be cured by appropriate treatment.

Treatment for therapy-resistant depressions

Various investigations have shown that only 70-80% of endogenous depressions respond to antidepressants administered by mouth. In a case where a patient with endogenous depression has failed to improve after treatment with two correctly selected antidepressants - each of which has been given for a period of three weeks in succession, in combination of course with psychotherapy - we then refer to the depression as therapy-resistant.
In such cases, the diagnosis of therapy-resistant depression should be checked by undertaking a renewed physical and psychic examination. Where the diagnosis of endogenous or exhaustion depression is then still found to be correct, and where

the depression exhibits strong overtones of anxiety, it has been our practice for the past eight years to administer intravenous drip infusions featuring a combination of clomipramine (Anafranil), which has a predominantly serotonergic effect, and maprotiline (Ludiomil), which has a predominantly noradrenergic effect, in 250 ml. of physiological saline. In cases of retarded, apathic depression showing lack of drive, we have been using for four years intravenous drip infusions containing nomifensine (1-3 ampoules of 25 mg.) in 250 ml. of physiological saline. With intravenous infusions of nomifensine (Alival) in cases of retarded endogenous depression, and with combined infusions of clomipramine (Anafranil) plus maprotiline (Ludiomil) in cases of endogenous depression with marked anxiety, we have succeeded in completely overcoming the resistance to therapy in 70% of the patients concerned.

Comparison of the results obtained with oral treatment and intravenous drip infusions has shown a statistically significant acceleration of the lifting of the depression with intravenous drip infusions.

FIGURE 13. Comparison of results obtained with oral and intravenous treatment for depression

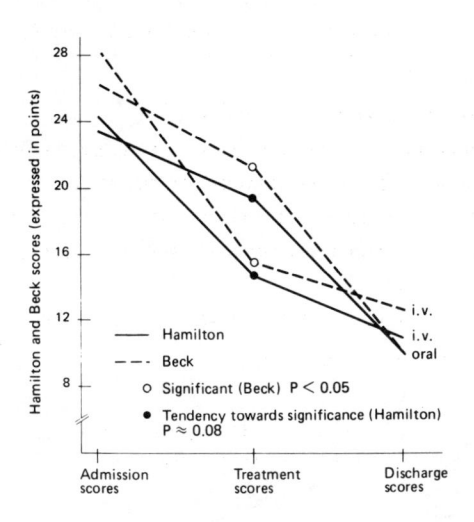

Comparison of results obtained with oral (N = 17) and intravenous (N = 15) treatment for depression

○ Significant (Beck) $P < 0.05$
● Tendency towards significance (Hamilton) $P \approx 0.08$

As Figure 13 clearly shows, even in therapy-resistant depressions intravenous infusions make it possible to achieve a marked lifting of the depression within 6-10 days. This treatment is easy to carry out and, provided there is no great danger of suicide, it can also be administered on an ambulant basis.

The WHO has planned a study, to be undertaken in various research centres throughout the world, in which oral and intravenous treatment for endogenous depressions is to be compared in a double-blind trial. If the results of this multicentre study confirm our findings, the question will then arise as to whether all endogenous depressions - and not simply the therapy-resistant ones - should not be treated right from the very beginning with intravenous infusions.

REFERENCES

Angst, J. (1961). A clinical analysis of the effects of tofranil in depression. Psychopharmacologia 2, 381-407.
Angst, J. (1963). Insidon als Antidepressivum. Nervenarzt 34, 76-80.
Berner, P. et al. (1973). Results of the enquiry in Vienna, Lower Austria, and the Burgenland. In Kielholz, P. (ed): Depression in everyday practice, Hans Huber, Berne.
Dilling, H. et al.(1978). Patienten mit psychischen Störungen in der Allgemeinpraxis und ihre psychiatrische Ueberweisungsbedürftigkeit. In: Häfner, H. (ed): Psychiatrische Epidemiologie, 135-160, Springer, Berlin.
Fazio, C. (1973): Enquiry on depression carried out in Italy in 1973. In:Kielholz, P. (ed): Depression in everyday practice, Hans Huber, Berne.
Freyhan, F.A. (1961). The influence of specific and non-specific factors and the clinical effects of psychotropic drugs. Neuropsychopharmacology 2, 189.
Freyhan, F.A. (1960). Die moderne psychiatrische Behandlung von Depresionen. Nervenarzt, 31, 112.
Hakim, C. (1973). Results of the enquiry in France. In: Kielholz, P. (ed): Depression in everyday practice, Hans Huber, Berne.
Helmchen, H. (1973). Results of the enquiry in the German Federal Republic and Berlin. In: Kielholz, P. (ed): Depression in everyday practice, Hans Huber, Berne.
Kielholz, P. (1973). Enquiries on depression in everyday practice. Results of the enquiry in Switzerland. In: Kielholz, P. (ed): Depression in everyday practice. Hans Huber, Berne.
Kielholz, P.,Gastpar, M. and Adams, C.(1978). Aspekte des Depressions-problems. Text zu einer Tonbildschau. Manuskript, Basel.
Kielholz, P., Ladewig, D. and Hauswirth, R. (1979). Psychische Störungen in der täglichen Praxis. Praxis, 68, 42, 1378-1382.

The Risks and Adverse Effects of ECT

R. E. Kendell

Department of Psychiatry, University of Edinburgh, Scotland, UK

ABSTRACT

Many laymen regard ECT as a dangerous treatment and it is usually depicted as such in films, plays and novels. In particular it is thought to have harmful effects on memory.
The available evidence, which is extensive, does not support this view. The risks of ECT are considerably less than those of untreated depression and probably less than those of tricyclic antidepressants. The risk of death is less than 1 in 20,000 treatments. There is no evidence, either from experimental ECS in animals or from postmortem brain histology in patients that ECT produces cerebral damage of any kind, but the convulsion is accompanied by a temporary increase in the permeability of the blood/brain barrier and occasional patients have one or two spontaneous grand mal fits after a course of treatment.
During and for a few weeks after a course of ECT the EEG is highly abnormal with bilateral delta waves and memory retention is impaired. This impairment of memory is the most important adverse effect of the treatment and is more severe with bilateral electrodes than with unilateral electrodes over the nondominant hemisphere. The results of two recent studies, using control groups and several different memory tests, strongly suggest that this impairment is purely temporary and that performance on all tests returns to normal within three, or at the most six, months of the end of treatment. Many patients, however, remain firmly convinced that their memories have never been quite the same since they had ECT. This may be because the temporary impairment caused by the treatment sensitises them to minor lapses of memory they would otherwise remain unaware of.

KEYWORDS

Electro-convulsive treatment; mortality; fractures; epilepsy; E.E.G. changes; memory impairment; depression.

The first and most important risk that has to be considered for any treatment is that of death itself. In this respect at least ECT, with or without a general anaesthetic, is surprisingly safe. Stensrud (1958) studied the mortality and neurological morbidity of a series of 893 women treated with unmodified ECT (or in a few cases chemically induced convulsions) at Gaustad Hospital in Norway in 1938-56. Although this population received a total of 24,562 treatments there were no deaths during or immediately after treatment and no patients were left with neurological deficits. There were three deaths within a few days of treatment but all three had pre-existing brain disease -Pick's disease, general paralysis and epilepsy/ mental deficiency. More recently Heshe and Roeder (1976) have studied the use of ECT in Denmark in the twelve month period from April 1972 to March 1973. 22,210 ECT were given, under general anaesthesia, in 3,438 courses, an average of 6.5 treatments to a course. Only one death was reported and the relationship of this to the treatment was doubtdul. The incidence of other side effects was also extremely low, and no higher when the anaesthetic was given by a psychiatrist or a nurse than when it was given by an anaesthetist. In England and Wales between 1957 and 1966 there were an average of 3.6 deaths/year associated with ECT but no estimate of the size of the population at risk is available (Granville-Grossman, 1971). Death when it does occur is usually due either to myocardial infarction or to the onset of a ventricular arthythmia, probably produced by vagal hyperactivity. The dangers of any treatment have, of course, to be set against those of the untreated illness and of alternative therapies and where ECT is concerned there is evidence that its introduction was associated with a steep fall in the hospital mortality of depressive illness (Slater, 1951). It has also been shown that the overall mortality of depressed patients over a three year period is lower in patients treated with ECT than in those treated with psychotherapy or small doses of antidepressant drugs (Avery & Winokur, 1976).
In the past fractures, mainly of mid thoracic vertebrae, and dislocations, particularly of the jaw, were a common complication, affecting up to 30% of patients in some series. Since suxamethonium came into routine use, however, complications of this kind have virtually ceased and even patients with serious spinal or other orthopaedic disorders can be given ECT with relative impunity.
The occurrence of sporadic grand mal fits for the first time in the weeks or months after a course of ECT has been reported several times (e.g. Blumenthal, 1955; Klotz, 1955; Stensrud, 1958). In many cases, though, the patients had either received other treatments like insulin coma therapy or tricyclic antidepressants which may have been partly or wholly responsible, or were known or suspected to have organic brain disease. In most of the early reports the patients had also received far longer courses of ECT than are normally given now. The analogy of the "kindling" phenomenon has recently revived interest in the relationship between ECT and epilepsy but a survey of 166 patients, who between them had received at least 2789 treatments, mostly in the previous two years, revealed only four people who had developed fits for the first time after ECT and in only two of these was in the likely cause (Blackwood, Cull, Freeman, Evans and Mawdsley, in press). There is general agreement that fits provoked by ECT rarely if ever persist for longer than a year, and so rarely require treatment.
A course of ECT almost invariably produces extensive EEG changes. If bilateral electrodes are used paroxysmal delta activity starts to appear in the frontal leads after the first two or three treatments and becomes steadily more prominent and extensive thereafter. A minority of patients also develop spike foci. This generalised delta activity wanes rapidly after the end of the course and in the majority of patients the EEG has returned to normal within three months (Klotz, 1955). In the past considerable interest was taken in the possibility that these dramatic changes might be different in responders and non-responders. There have been claims, for example, that responders develop widespread delta activity at an earlier stage (Fink and Kahn, 1957), or show a greater increase in spectral energy in the 9-12 Hz range (Kurland, Turek, Brown an Wagman, 1976), or that delta activity is

more rapidly extinguished by thiopentone in those who subsequently relapse (Roth, Kay, Shaw and Green, 1957) but none of these relationships has ever been confirmed. Whether ECT ever produces enduring EEG changes, and if so under what circumstances, is currently being studies by Sainsbury and his colleagues in Chichester.
The common immediate side effects of ECT are headache, confusion and memory disturbance, though the headache and confusion are usually mild and last only an hour or two. Impairment of memory is invariably present if appropriate testing is done, though many patients remain unaware of it. In a recent survey of a representative group of 166 patients the commonest side effects recorded in medical or nursing notes were headache (16%), confusion (9%) and memory disturbance (7%) (Freeman and Kendell, 1980). A rather different picture emerged, however, when the same patients were asked a year later about the side effects they remembered. 20% could remember none, but 64% reported some impairment of memory, and 48% remembered having a headache and 27% feeling confused on at least one occasion, though in most cases these symptoms were relatively mild. Occasional patients also complain of nausea or vomiting, clumsiness, or muscle pains induced by suxamethonium.
The short term memory impairment produced by ECT has been studied many times. There is both a retrograde component, most noticeable for recent events, and also difficulty in retaining newly acquired information. It is well established that this memory impairment and the associated confusion are both less severe and more short-lived when ECT is given unilaterally to the non-dominant hemisphere than when bilateral electrodes are used (Heshe, Roder and Theilgaard, 1978). It is also well established that if the electrodes are placed over the non-dominant hemisphere there is a selective impairment of non-verbal learning, and a selective impairment of verbal learning if they are placed over the dominant hemisphere (Halliday, Davison, Browne and Kreeger, 1968; Squire and Slater, 1978). These disturbances wane rapidly after the end of treatment in the same way as the EEG changes described above. It is not entirely clear, however, how long they may persist, or whether patients are ever left with an enduring memory deficit, though these are obviously crucial questions. Transient impairement of memory for a few weeks is usually no more important or distressing than a dry mouth or many of the other common side effects of drug treatments. A lasting memory impairment restricted to events taking place at the time of treatment would also be relatively unimportant. Indeed many people might be glad to have a rather hazy memory of a painful and distressing illness. But a permanently impaired ability to recall more distant events or, worse still, to register new information subsequently, would be much more serious and a powerful objection to the treatment.
Although most investigations have failed to find any evidence of lasting impairment there are one or two reports which at least raise the possibility of a permanent deficit. Janis (1950) interviewed nineteen patients before starting treatment to obtain detailed information about events, important and trivial, pleasand and unpleasant, in their past lives. When he re-interviewed them approximately four weeks after the end of the course all nineteen were unable to recall some of the memories they had described in the pretreatment interview, and in the five patients re-interviewed six to ten weeks later most of these deficits were still present. Eleven control patients, matched for age and education, were also interviewed on two occasions the same interval apart but in them memory lapses were almost non-existent. The majority of both groups were schizophrenics and the ECT group received an average of 17 unmodified treatments at a rate of three/week, i.e. a considerably langer number and at a higher rate than is normal nowadays. More recently, Halliday et al. (1968) have reported a comparison of the differential effects of bilateral and left and right unilateral electrode placements in which nonverbal memory had not returned to its pretreatment level in the bilateral group at final testing, or verbal memory in the left unilateral (dominant hemisphere) group. Because their main interest lay elsewhere the authors themselves paid little attention to these findings. From the information they provide, however, it appears that delayed non-verbal learning in the bilateral electrodes group was the only test score significantly worse three months after treatment

than before, and then only at the 5% confidence level with a one-tailed t test. Moreover, twenty of the 44 patients retested at three months had had an average of four furhter ECT in the interim, so the interval after the last treatment would actually have been less than three months.

Assessment of most of the other studies in the literature is complicated by the fact that severe depression itself produces extensive cognitive impairment, though it is mainly the registration rather than the retention of memory that is affected (Sternberg and Jarvik, 1976). It is not sufficient, therefore, to demonstrate that memory is as good or better after a course of ECT than it was immediately beforehand. This may only mean that impairment from depression has been replaced by impairment from ECT. For this reason studies based only on a comparison of cognitive performance immediately before and a few weeks after ECT, like that of Cronholm and Molander (1964), cannot be conclusive. A further problem is that several studies, like that of Turek and Block (1974), have relied on the Weschler Memory Scale, which is a measure of registration rather than of retention, as their main or only index of impairment.

To be sure of detecting any persistent congnitive deficit that might be present it is essential, therefore, to test all aspects of memory, and also to have an estimate of cognitive function before ECT that is uncontaminated by the effect of depression. As it is not feasible to test people before they become depressed, and unethical to give ECT to non-patients, this means that a control group is essential, composed either of normal people or of depressives who have recovered without ECT. A few of the older studies, like that of Korin, Fink and Kwalwasser(1956) did employ a control group, but only used a restricted range of tests. These authors tested recall of word lists, immediately and after ten minutes, at weekly intervals in a diagnostically heterogeneous group of 40 patients who received 12 ECT in five weeks, and also in 21 matched controls. Learning initially deteriorated in the ECT group, but three weeks after the end of the course it was better than it had been before treatment started, and also better than in the controls (presumably because the clinical condition of the controls had not improved so much).

Two more recent studies have used a much wider range of tests as well as a control group. Squire and Chase (1975) tested 16 patients who had received bilateral and 10 who had received unilateral ECT six to nine months before, and 12 control patients who had never had ECT. All 38 were visited at home on three occasions and given six different tests of delayed retention and remote memory, involving verbal, visual and casual learning. No significant differences were found on any of the six tests. However, 63% of the bilateral ECT patients, but only 30% of the unilateral patients and 17% of the controls, were convinced that their memories were worse than they had been previously. As the test scores of those with memory complaints wereno different from those without complaints Squire and Chace were forced to conclude either that ECT, particularly bilateral ECT, causes an enduring memory impairment too subtle to be detected by the tests they used or, alternatively, that the marked temporary impairment produced by the treatment makes parients sensitive to "normal" memory lapses they would otherwise disregard.

A large prospective study has recently been reported from Edinburgh by Weeks, Freeman and Kendell (1980). These authors gave a battery of 19 tests covering an unusually wide range of cognitive functions to 51 depressives before they received ECT and again one week, three months and six months after the end of the course. The same tests were given to 51 control patients, matched for age, social class, educational attainment and severity of depression, who did not receive ECT. The ECT patients received an average of 7.2 treatments, 15 with unilateral and 36 with bilateral electrodes, and by good fortune there were no significant differences in the types or qualities of antidepressant drugs received by the two groups. Partly because their initial performance was impaired by depression, the ECT patients did not score worse on any test one week after the end of their course than they had done before starting. Indeed, their performance on several tests was significantly improved. Three months after treatment there were significant

differences between the ECT and non-ECT groups on only two of the 19 tests. The ECT patients were unable to remember the names of famous personalities from the decade 1970-79 as well as the controls, but performed significantly **better** on a test of ability to shift mental set. Six months after treatment there was only one significant difference, the ECT group performing significantly **better** than the controls on the Logical Memory Test.
Scores on the same test battery were also obtained for 130 normal volunteers. 51 members of this population were matched with the ECT patients for age, sex, social class and educational attainment and their scores compared. Six months after the end of treatment both patients groups (ECT and non-ECT) scored lower than these normal subjects on several tests, but Weeks and his colleagues attributed these modest deficits either to the residual depressive symptoms of the two patient groups, or to the psychotropic medication they were still receiving.
Taken in isolation these results strongly suggest that the temporary cognitive impairments produced by ECT have disappeared completely by six months after the end of treatment, and probably by three months. However, the same authors also studied a group of 26 people, mainly identified by a newspaper appeal, who had received ECT in the past and were convinced that it had permanently harmed them in some way (Freeman, Weeks and Kendell, 1980). Most of these people had complaints about their memory; either that they had gaps in their memory for events which had taken place months or years before they had ECT; or that since receiving ECT they had more difficulty remembering names, messages, phone numbers etc. When they were given the same battery of 19 tests that had been used in the prospective study described above their scores on seven of the 19 were significantly worse than those of a group of 53 matched controls. The ECT complainers had more depressive symptoms than the controls, and more were currently taking psychotropic drugs, but analysis of variance/covariance suggested that only part of their deficit in cognitive performance could be explained by these differences. The authors were left, therefore, much as Squire and Chase had been, with two alternative explanations for their results: either ECT had, as the subjects themselves believed, produced mild but detectable memory impairment; Or, alternatively, ECT was being blamed inappropriately for a mild deterioration arising for some other reason because its initial effects on memory made it a plausible culprit.
In summary, there is still no firm evidence that the cognitive impairments produced by ECT are ever permanent, but the possibility cannot be excluded and the suspicion must remain. Indeed, 41% of the 3000 psychiatrists who responded to the American Psychiatric Association's recent questionnaire endorsed the statement "It is likely that ECT produces slight or subtle brain damage" and only 26% disagreed (American Psychiatric Association, 1978). Some of the reasons why the issue was not decided long ago have already been referred to. Depression itself affects memory, particularly retention, so in the short term any impairment produced by ECT is likely to be masked by recovery from depression, while in the long term poor performance may be due to the persistence or recurrence of mild depressive symptoms or to the effects of current medication rather than to previous ECT. Perhaps the most important problem of all, however, is the ubiquity of complaints of poor memory, and the poor relationship between these complaints and objective evidence of impairment. In a recent study of a mixed population of elderly psychiatric patients and their relatives 76% of all subjects complained about their memories, but these complaints correlated with depressive symptoms rather than with objective impairment (Kahn, Zarit, Hilbert and Niederehe, 1975). Indeed, for some tests there was a significant negative correlation between subjective complaint and objective deficit!
Despite early reports of cerebral oedema, neuronal degeneration, gliosis and petechial haemorrhages in the midbrain there is no evidence either from experimental ECS in laboratory animals or histological studies of patients' brains that electrically induced convulsions produce cerebral damage of any kind unless very large numbers of shocks are given in a short space of time. There is evidence, however,

of a temporary breakdown of the so-calles "blood/brain barrier". Using horseradish peroxidase as marker substance Bolwing, Hertz and Westergaard (1977) showed that even a single ECS produced staining of brain tissue in some animals. This was abolished, however, by transection of the cervical cord, suggesting that this increased permeability is secondary to the rise in blood pressure accompanying the convulsion. Bolwing and Hertz also showed that the permeability of the blood brain barrier to small molecules increased temporarily in psychiatric patients receiving ECT (Bolwing, Hertz, Paulson, Spotoft and Rafaelsen, 1977). However, as similar changes in both permeability and cerebral blood flow were produced simply by breathing 3% CO_2 they concluded that the increased permeability was probably secondary to increased blood flow in both cases, either because of a stretching of endothelial cells in cerebral vessels or the opening of new capillaries.
Hamilton, Stocker and Spencer (1979) have recently claimed that the temporary impairment of cognitive function associated with ECT correlates highly with the magnitude of the associated rise in blood pressure. If confirmed this is potentially important, because it suggests that the cognitive impairment may also be secondary to increased permeability of the blood/brain barrier, and possibly preventable by drugs which abolish or reduce the rise in blood pressure.

REFERENCES

American Psychiatric Association (1978) Electroconvulsive Therapy: Report of the Task Force on Electroconvulsive Therapy of the American Psychiatric Association. Task Force Report 14. Washington D.C.
Avery, D. and G. Winokur (1976). Mortality in depressed patients treated with electroconvulsive therapy and antidepressants. Archives of General Psychiatry, 33, 1029-37.
Blackwood, D.H.R., R. Cull, C.P.L. Freeman, J.I. Evans and C. Mawdsley. A study of the incidence of epilepsy following ECT. Journal of Neurology, Neurosurgery and Psychiatry. (In press).
Blumenthal, I.J. (1955). Spontaneous seizures and related encephalographic findings following shock therapy. Journal of Nervous and Mental Disease, 122, 581-8.
Bolwing, T.G., M.M. Hertz, O.B. Paulson, H. Spotoft and O.J. Rafaelsen (1977). The permeability of the blood-brain barrier during electrically induced seizures in man. European Journal of Clinical Investigation, 7, 87-93.
Bolwing, T.G., M.M. Hertz and E. Westergaard (1977). Acute hypertension causing blood-brain barrier breakdown during epileptic seizures. Acta Neurologica Scandinavica, 56, 335-42.
Cronholm, B. and L. Molander (1964). Memory disturbances after electroconvulsive therapy. Acta Psychiatrica Scandinavica, 40, 212-6.
Fink, M. and R.L. Kahn (1957). Relation of electro-encephalographic delta activity to behavioural response in electroshock. Archives of Neurology and Psychiatry, 78, 516-25.
Freeman, C.P. and R.E. Kendell (1980). ECT: Patients' experiences and attitudes. British Journal of Psychiatry, 137, 8-16.
Freeman, C.P.L., D. Weeks, and R.E. Kendell (1980). ECT: Patients who complain. British Journal of Psychiatry, 137, 17-25.
Granville-Grossman, K. (1971). Physical treatments of affective disorders. In Recent Advances in Clinical Psychiatry, p. 13. London: J. & A. Churchill.
Halliday, A.M., K. Davison, M.W. Browne, and L.C. Kreeger (1968). A comparison of the effects on depression and memory of bilateral E.C.T. and unilateral E.C.T. to the dominant and non-dominant hemispheres. British Journal of Psychiatry, 114, 997-1012.
Hamilton, M., M.J. Stocker and C.M. Spencer (1979). Post ECT cognitive defect and elevation of blood pressure. British Journal of Psychiatry, 135, 77-8.
Heshe, J. and E. Roeder (1976). Electroconvulsive therapy in Denmark. British Journal of Psychiatry, 128, 241-5.
Heshe, J., E. Röder and A. Theilgaard (1978). Unilateral and bilateral ECT. Acta Psychiatrica Scandinavica, Suppl 275.
Janis, I.L. (1950). Psychologic effects of electir convulsive treatments. Journal of Nervous and Mental Disease, 111, 359-82.
Kahn, R.L., S.H. Zarit, N.M. Hilbert and G. Niederehe (1975). Memory complaint and impairment in the aged. Archives of General Psychiatry, 32, 1569-73.
Klotz, M. (1955). Serial electroencephalographic changes due to electrotherapy. Diseases of the Nervous System, 16, 120-1.
Korin, H., M. Fink, and S. Kwalwasser (1956). Relation of changes in memory and learning to improvement in electroshock. Confinia Neurologica, 16, 88-96.
Kurland, A.A., I.S. Turek, C.C. Brown and A.M.I. Wagman (1976). Electroconvulsive therapy and EEG correlates in depressive disorders. Comprehensive Psychiatry, 17, 581-9.
Roth, M., D.W.K. Kay, J. Shaw and J. Green (1957). Prognosis and pentothal induced electroencephalographic changes in electroconvulsive treatment. Electroencephalography and Clinical Neurophysiology, 9, 225-37.
Slater, E.T.O. (1951). Evaluation of electric convulsion therapy as compared with conservative methods of treatment in depressive states. Journal of Mental Science, 97, 567-9.

Squire, L.R. and P.M. Chase (1975). Memory functions six to nine months after electroconvulsive therapy. Archives of General Psychiatry, 32, 1557-64.
Squire, L.R. and P.C. Slater (1978). Bilateral and unilateral ECT: effects on verbal and non-verbal memory. American Journal of Psychiatry, 135, 1316-20.
Stensrud, P.A. (1958). Cerebral complications following 24, 562 convulsion treatments in 893 patients. Acta Psychiatrica et Neurologica Scandinavica, 33, 115-26.
Sternberg, D.E. and M.E. Jarvik (1976). Memory functions in depression. Archives of General Psychiatry, 33, 219-24.
Turek, I.S. and B. Block (1974) Memory changes with ECT in depression. British Journal of Clinical Practice, 28, 94-5.
Weeks, D., C.P.L. Freeman and R.E. Kendell (1980) ECT: Enduring cognitive deficits? British Journal of Psychiatry, 137, 26-37.

Psychometric, Electroencephalographic and Histochemical Changes Following Long-term Lithium Administration. Preliminary Observations

G. N. Christodoulou, G. N. Papadimitriou, A. Kokkevi,
S. Malliara-Loulakaki, M. R. Issidorides,
M. T. Panayiotakopoulou

Department of Psychiatry, University of Athens, Eginition Hospital, Athens, Greece

ABSTRACT

Twelve manic-depressive patients treated with lithium prophylactically were inv
stigated psychometrically (memory function), electroencephalographically and hi
stochemically (blood cells)prior to, 2 and 12 months after initiation of treatm
The findings revealed in the majority of patients some degree of memory dysfunc
EEG abnormalities and qualitative changes in the peripheral blood eosinophils.

KEY WORDS

Lithium, manic-depressive psychosis, memory, psychometrics, electroencephalogra
histochemistry.

INTRODUCTION

This preliminary report deals with psychometric, electroencephalographic (EEG)
histochemical findings obtained prior to and following long-term administration
lithium to patients with recurrent affective disorders.
The aim of the psychometric study was to further investigate the effect of lith
on memory. As shown by previous investigations lithium produces memory disturba
in normal controls (Schou, 1968, Kropf and Müller-Oerlinghausen, 1979) patients
with Huntington's chorea (Aminoff, and co-workers, 1974) and laboratory animals
(Mark and Watts, 1971; Johnson, 1976). Also there are some data which indicate
that lithium produces memory dysfunction in manic-depressive patients (Christod
lou, Siafakas and Rinieris, 1977; Christodoulou and co-workers, 1978; Kusumo ar
Vaughan 1977; Christodoulou and co-workers, 1981), although the existing evider
for such an action is not shared by all investigators (Telford and Worrall, 19.
Kjellman, Karlberg and Thorell, 1980).
The aim of the EEG study was to further explore the issue of lithium-induced EI
changes and to correlate the findings with those revealed by the psychometric
tests.
Finally, the aim of the histochemical investigation was to confirm previous obs
vations (Issidorides and co-workers, 1981) which indicate that lithium produces
qualitative changes in the blood leukocytes in addition to its well known quant
tative effect (Mayfield and Brown, 1966).

MATERIAL AND METHODS

Seventeen manic-depressive patients in normothymia (9 men, 8 women, age range 21 to 69 years (mean 41.52+13.97), duration of illness 0,5 to 36 years (mean 13.44+ 9.50) participated in the study (Table 1).

TABLE 1. Clinical and Laboratory Data of Patients During Lithium Psychoprophylaxis

Subject	Age(years) and Sex	Duration of Illness (years)	Duration of Lithium Treatment (months)	Range of Lithium daily dosage(mg)	Range of plasma Lithium levels (mEq/l)
1	22 F	5	12	900-1500	0,55-1,05
2	23 F* Δ	2	12	900-1200	0,28-0,70
3	37 F Δ	19	12	900-1500	0,27-1,00
4	57 F Δ	36	12	900-1200	0,68-1,50
5	69 F*	8	12	900-1200	0,28-0,74
6	41 M*	19	12	900-1500	0,46-1,10
7	40 M*	10	12	900-1500	0,32-0,98
8	29 M	4	12	900-1500	0,40-1,30
9	60 F*	21	12	900	0,60-1,00
10	34 F	2	12	900-1500	0,57-1,02
11	39 M*	13	12	900-1500	0,52-0,78
12	53 M	24	11	900	0,60-0,90
13	21 M	0,5	12	900-1200	0,60-1,00
14	50 M	12	10	900-1800	0,48-1,15
15	35 F	17	8	900-1200	0,62-1,25
16	42 M	21	8	900-1200	0,68-1,08
17	54 M*	15	6	900-1200	0,58-0,82

* Positive family history
Δ Thyrohormone

All patients were euthyroid. Three women were under thyrohormone treatment.
All patients were drug-free for 15 days and had not received ECT for at least 6 months before onset of the study.
Mean daily dosage of lithium ranged from 900 to 1800 mg and plasma lithium levels ranged from 0,27 to 1,50 mEq/l.
Our patients were submitted to the usual laboratory tests as well as to psychometric tests, EEG investigation and histochemical study before, after 2 and after 12 months following onset of psychoprophylactic administration of lithium.
The following psychometric tests were administered:
a) Rey's Auditory-Verbal Learning test (Rey, 1964).
b) The Associate Learning test of the Wechsler Memory Scale (Wechsler, 1945).
c) Benton's Visual Retention test (Benton, 1963).
d) The Digit Span Subtest of the WAIS (Wechsler, 1968).
Description of administered tests
a) Rey's Auditory - Verbal Learning test:
A list of 15 words is read to the subject at the rate of one per second and he is asked to repeat as many words as he can remember. There are three successive trials. The score consists of the number of words correctly recalled. Two different lists of words of similar difficulty were given at each examination.

b) The Associate Learning task of the Wechsler Memory Scale:
A list of ten word-pairs was read to the subject and he was asked to give the second pair of each couple after presentation of the test pair. There are three successive trials. The score consists of the number of words correctly recalled. Two lists of different words of similar difficulty were administered at each examination.
c) Benton's Visual Retention test:
1. Each card of the test was exposed for 10 seconds and the subject was asked to draw the designs immediately after their presentation (immediate retention task).
2. Each card was exposed for 10 seconds and the subject was asked to draw the designs after a 15 seconds' delay (delayed retention task). The score consists of the number of errors.
d) The Digit Span Subtest of the WAIS:
The subject was asked to repeat orally presented series of digits, forwards and backwards. The score consists of the number of digits correctly repeated forwards and backwards.
The EEG investigation consisted of three routine EEGs. The first EEG was taken before onset of treatment, the second EEG two months and the third EEG twelve months after onset of treatment. An Elema Schönander 16-Channel Electroencephalograph was used.
Blood smears for the histochemical study were obtained at the same time intervals as above, fixed in 10% formalin and stained with the Mallory Trichrome differential (Issidorides and co-workers, 1981).

RESULTS

From our original sample of 17 patients, 12 completed one year of continuous lithium ingestion and were therefore included in this study. These patients were 7 women and 5 men, had an age range of 21 to 69 (mean 39,33+15,5) and the duration of the patients' illnesses ranged from 0,5 to 36 years (mean 11,6+10,5).
Table 2 shows the results of the psychometric and the EEG investigation. As indicated in this table, 7 out of 11 patients were assessed as having developed memory disturbances at 2 months and 8 patients at 12 months after initiation of treatment. One of the patients was not included in the psychometric investigation because of his very low I.Q.

TABLE 2. Results

Age(years) and Sex	Duration of illness (years)	Lithium daily dosage (mg) At 2 months	Lithium daily dosage (mg) At 12 months	Plasma Lithium levels (mEq/l) At 2 months	Plasma Lithium levels (mEq/l) At 12 months	Side - effects Memory A	Side - effects Memory B_{vsA}	Side - effects Memory C_{vsA}	Side - effects EEG A	Side - effects EEG B	Side - effects EEG C
22 F	5	900	1500	0,55	0,88	−	+	−	+	+	
23 F*Δ	2	1200	1200	0,40	0,55	+	+	+	+	+	
37 F Δ	19	1200	1500	0,77	0,98	+	+	+	+	+	
57 F Δ	36	900	900	1,00	1,03	+	+	+	+	+	
69 F*	8	900	1200	0,40	0,64	+	+	+	+	+	
60 F*	21	900	900	1,00	0,80	−	−	+	+	+	
34 F	2	1200	1500	0,62	1,02	−	−	+	+	+	
41 M*	19	1500	1500	1,10	0,72	−	−	−	−	+	
40 M*	10	1200	1500	0,68	0,80	+	+	−	+	+	
29 M	4	1200	1200	0,90	0,96	+	+	−	−	+	
39 M*	13	1200	1500	0,58	0,58	+	+	+	+	−	
21 M	0,5	1200	1200	1,00	0,87			−	−	−	

* Positive family history
Δ Thyrohormone

A: Prior to initiation of Li
B: 2 months after initiation of Li
C: 12 months after initiation of Li

It should be noted, however, that memory disturbances were not revealed by all administered tests. In 4 of our 11 patients memory performance deteriorated in Benton's visual retention test and in two of the above patients the Associate Learning test of the Wechsler Memory Scale also showed impaired performance. Three more patients had impaired performance only in the digit span sub-test of the WAIS and two in Rey's test.

With respect to the EEG findings, as shown in table II, 10 out of 12 investigated patients had abnormal records 12 months after initiation of treatment. It should be noted however, that the records of 6 of these patients were already abnormal before initiation of treatment. Also, the EEG record of one patient improved following 12 months' treatment. The most frequently observed EEG abnormalities were bursts of paroxysmal slow waves with occasional spiky formations or sharp waves (with or without lateralization).

With one exception, in all patients the histochemical investigation revealed findings illustrated in figure I.

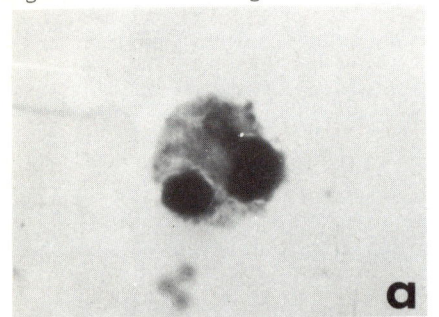

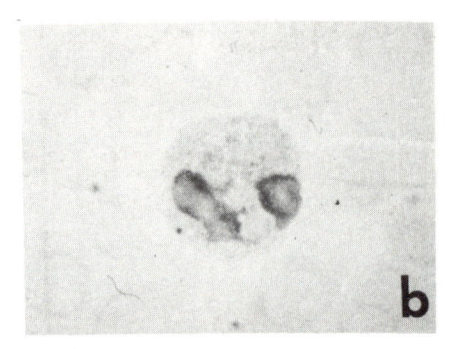

FIGURE I. Eosinophils of a manic-depressive patient. Drug-free state (a), and one year after initiation of lithium treatment (b). Mallory's differential stain.

Figure I shows eosinophils of one of our manic-depressive patients in the drug-free state (fig. 1a) and one year after initiation of lithium treatment (fig. 1b) stained with Mallory's differential stain. This procedure combines three acidic stains (Acid fuchsin, Orange G, Aniline blue) which react with basic proteins. We observed that the two factors which characterize these granulocytes in the drug-free manic-depressive patients, i.e. red fuchsinophilic, loosely condensed nuclear chromatin and disrupted leaky cytoplasmic granules, were modified by the drug. The nuclear chromatin reacted yellow with Orange G, which has affinity for its condensed form, and the granules became totally unreactive (fig. 1b).

DISCUSSION

The data of the present preliminary report support our previous findings which indicate that lithium may produce some degree of memory dysfunction in manic-depressive patients (Christodoulou and co-workers, 1981). Squire and co-workers, 1980, who studied the effect of lithium on memory in 16 psychiatric patients who received lithium for 2 weeks, noted that lithium did not significantly affect performance on formal tests of memory. These authors state that it is possible that "measurable effects of lithium on memory would have appeared if treatment had been continued longer than two weeks". This is a possibility that should be considered in view of the fact that our own patients were assessed after a much longer period of lithium administration. It should, however, be pointed out that only one of our four patients who had not developed memory trouble at two months developed such a side-effect at 12 months. The other three patients' memory function was unaffected.

Our EEG findings confirmed previous publications which indicate that lithium pro-

duces a variety of nonspecific abnormalities of the bioelectrical activity of the brain.
It is interesting to note that half of the manic-depressive patients of our sample had abnormal EEG records to begin with. This is not in keeping with the prevalent impression that manic-depressives have essentially similar EEGs to controls.
It is perhaps of some significance that all three patients who were on thyrohormone showed abnormalitites both in their memory function and in their EEG records. This probably indicates that thyrohormone administered either alone or in conjunction with lithium may produce psycho-organic phenomena, either manifest or subclinical. Further observations are clearly needed in order to confirm this possibility.
A positive family history may have some relevance to our findings since 4 of our 6 patients with positive family history manifested both memory disturbances and EEG abnormalities 2 and 12 months after initiation of lithium treatment. On the contrary age, sex, duration of illness, lithium daily dosage and plasma lithium levels seem to be unrelated to either memory disturbances or EEG findings.
The histochemical study confirmed our original observations in a smaller group of patients (Issidorides and co-workers, 1981),which indicate that lithium produces beneficial qualitative changes in the blood eosinophils of manic-depressive patients which are abnormal prior to drug-treatment. These results are attributed to the property of the lithium ion to cause conformational changes in nuclear and cytoplasmic proteins (Bunney and co-workers, 1979), presumably affecting their function.-

REFERENCES

Aminoff, M.S., and J. Marshall (1974). Lancet, i, 107.
Benton, A.L. (1963). The revised visual retention test, New York, The Psychological Corporation.
Bunney, W.E. Jr., A. Pert, J. Rosenblatt, C.B. Pert, and D. Galloper (1979). Arch Gen. Psychiat. 36, 898-901.
Christodoulou, G.N., Siafakas, A., and P.M. Rinieris (1977). Acta Psychiat.Belg., 77, 260-266.
Christodoulou, G.N., A. Kokkevi, E.P. Lykouras and C.N. Stefanis (1978). IInd World Congress of Biological Psychiatry, Barcelona, Spain.
Christodoulou, G.N., A. Kokkevi, E.P. Lykouras, C.N. Stefanis, and G.N. Papadimitriou (1981). Am. J. Psychiatry (in press)
Johnson, F.N. (1976). Br. J. Pharmacol. 56, 87-90.
Issidorides, M.R., E.P. Lykouras, G.N. Papadimitriou, M.T. Panayiotakopoulou, and G.N. Christodoulou (1981). Histochemical changes in peripheral blood leukocytes during lithium treatment. In G.N. Christodoulou (editor): Aspects of Preventive Psychiatry, Karger, Basel (in press).
Kjellman, B.F., B.E. Karlberg, and L.-H. Thorell (1980). Acta Psychiat. Scand.,62, 32-46.
Kropf, D., and B. Müller-Oerlinghausen (1979). Acta Psychiat. Scand. 59, 97-124.
Kusumo, K.S., and M. Vaughan (I977). Br. J. Psychiatry, 131, 453-457.
Mark, R.F., and M.E. Watts (1971). Proc. Roy. Soc. Med., 178, 439-454.
Mayfield, D., and R.C. Brown (1966). J. Psychiat. Res. 4, 207-219.
Rey, A. (1964). L'examen clinique en Psychologie. Paris, Presses Universitaires de France.
Squire, L.R., L.L. Judd, D.S. Janowsky, and L.H. Huey (1980). Am. J. Psychiatry, 137, 1042-1046.
Schou, M. (1968). J. Psychiat. Res., 6, 67-95.
Telford, R., and E.P. Worrall (1978). Br. J. Psychiatry, 133, 424-428.
Wechsler, D. (1945). J. Psychol. 19, 87-95
Wechsler, D. (1958). The measurement and appraisal of adult intelligence. Williams and Wilkins, Baltimore, p 70.

Sleep Deprivation in the Prophylaxis of Manic-depressive Illness

G. N. Christodoulou, G. N. Papadimitriou, E. P. Lykouras,
C. N. Stefanis, D. E. Malliaras and G. M. Trikkas

Department of Psychiatry, University of Athens, Eginition Hospital, Athens, Greece

ABSTRACT

The existing methods of prophylaxis of the recurrent affective disorders, namely lithium, maintenance treatment with tricyclic compounds, prophylaclic ECT and prophylactic administration of 5-HTP are critically reviewed.
Data indicating that, in addition to its therapeutic value, sleep deprivation can also exercise a prophylactic effect in both unipolar and bipolar patients are presented.
The above findings suggest that this method may prove to be of first choice in "rapid cyclers", a sub-group of manic-depressive patients who don't seem to benefit from lithium treatment.

KEYWORDS

Sleep deprivation; manic-depressive psychosis; psychoprophylaxis; affective disorders.

INTRODUCTION

The aims of this paper are threefold. First, to critically evaluate the existing biological methods of prophylaxis of the recurrent affective disorders. Second, to briefly review the evidence concerning the effectiveness of therapeutic sleep deprivation (S.D.) in depression. And third, to review the existing data pertaining to the response of manic-depressive patients to prophylactic sleep deprivation (P.S.D.)

Psychoprophylaxis of the recurrent affective disorders

Various methods of prophylaxis of manic-depressive psychosis have at times been suggested. Among them lithium is undoubtedly an effective, widely used and "global" method (in that its effectiveness applies to both the depressive and the manic phase of the illness). Additionally, contrary to other methods of prophylaxis which have not been thoroughly evaluated, adequate experience has accumulated on the effectiveness, indications and undesirable effects of lithium.
It should be pointed out, however, that certain categories of manic-depressive patients (e.g. "rapid cyclers") do not seem to respond to prophylactic lithium (Dun-

ner and Fieve, 1974). Other patients cannot be even tried on lithium because of
their poor physical condition, particularly serious kidney dysfunction but also
serious thyroid and cardiac dysfunctions. Also, there is a third category of patients who find it difficult to conform with the procedure associated with lithium
therapy (regular lithium measurements, clinical follow-up, kidney function tests,
etc) particularly when their motivation is poor (often due to a mild, sub-clinical
depression) or they live in remote rural areas lacking the necessary laboratory
facilities.
It is thus apparent that there is place for alternative methods of prophylaxis.
Tricyclic anti-depressants have been found effective in the prevention of recurrences of endogenous depression (Seager and Bird,1962; Imlah and collaborators, 1965:
Mindham, 1981). This method, however, has the limitation of being effective only
in unipolar depression and not in bipolar affective disorder (Prien, Klett and Caffey, 1973). The cardiotoxic effect of the tricyclic drugs, which has been reported
to be responsible for sudden deaths (Coull and collaborators, 1971) should also be
taken into consideration (Boston collaborative drug surveillance program, 1972) as
well as their unpleasant autonomic side-effects.
Even before the lithium era, Stevenson and Geoghegan (1951) had suggested that
montly ECT could exercise a prophylactic effect in manic-depressive patients. However, long-term follow-up studies have not been conducted and the effectiveness of
this method has not been replicated. Besides, submitting a person in mormothymia
to prophylactic ECT would be more than problematic, in view of the notorious unpopularity of this method.
Van Praag and de Haan (1980) suggested that 5-HTP (a 5-HT precursor) reduces the
relapse rate of endogenous vital depressions and that this effect appears to be more pronounced in patients whose disorder of central 5-HT metabolism is more persistent. More research is needed in order to confirm this interesting possibility.

Therapeutic sleep deprivation

Sleep deprivation (S.D.) has been shown by a number of investigators to be therapeutically effective in depressive patients (Pflug and Tölle, 1971; Bhanji and
Roy, 1975; Larsen, Hingberg and Skovgaard, 1976 and others).
In a review of 10 studies Roy and Bhanji (1976) have concluded that this method
may be a useful treatment in a third to a half of patients with endogenous depression and a bibliography search by Post, Gillin and Bunney (1979) revealed that a
usually transient antidepressant effect occurs in one-third to two-thirds of medication-free depressed patients. Our own observations are in keeping with this
general impression. Out of 16 drug-free endogenous depressive patients (12 female,
4 male) treated therapeutically with two 36 hours' total sleep deprivation sessions per week, six patients (five female, one male) responded to treatment (unpublished data). Bhanji, Roy and Baulieu (1978) identified two groups of responders
differing in term of self-reported emotional arousal during the course of the
sleepless night. Patients of the first group improved during the day following S.D.
whilst those of the second group did not respond until after the next night's sleep.
Vogel and collaborators (1980) have drawn attention to the beneficial effect of
REM sleep deprivation in depression and Schilgen and Tölle (1978) have reported
improvement of depressive patients with partial sleep deprivation (awakening of
the patients during the second half of the night).
As refers to the profile of the responder there seems to be a consensus that a positive response is associated with severe endogenous depression. On the contrary,
sex, length of illness, age and the unipolar-bipolar distinction don't seem to be
of any predictive value (for review see Gerner and collaborators, 1979).

Prophylactic sleep deprivation

Very limited research has been conducted on the issue of S.D. prophylaxis.
The case of a female unipolar depressive "rapid cycler" who showed a spectacular
response to prophylactic S.D. has been reported by our team (Christodoulou and col-

laborators, 1978a). Before initiation of S.D. treatment this patient had 15 attacks of depression (three of them accompanied by serious suicidal attempts) occurring once a month and lasting 6-10 days. After initiation of S.D. therapy the patient remained depression-free for a period of 8 months, 2 weeks. During this period she should "normally" have had at least 8 attacks. It is worth noting that the patient was tried on lithium and tricyclics with negative results. Follow-up revealed that whenever she attempted to discontinue prophylactic S.D., severe depressive bouts followed. Unfortunately the last of these bouts was accompanied by suicidal ideation and the patient eventually committed suicide. At that stage we considered the possibility of precipitation of the patient's fatal outcome by sleep deprivation particularly since a Scandinavian patient reported by Rasmussen (1978) had also committed suicide after treatment with S.D. Yet, none of our patients who were later theated with S.D. had a similar evolution of their illness.
Kjellman, Larsson and Thorell (1977) in a Congress report have presented a pilot study demonstrating the beneficial prophylactic effect of S.D. in two "rapid cyclers", one male patient of 54 and one female patient of 67. The first patient had not responded to lithium and the second patient had discontinued treatment due to side-effects. The frequency of S.D. sessions was originally one per week but later on it progressively descreased.
The beneficial effect of prophylactic weekly 36 hours' total sleep deprivation in the case of two female patients (one recurrent depressive "rapid cycler" and one manic-depressive patient) was subsequently reported by our team (Christodoulou and collaborators, 1978b).
In an effort to draw some general conclusions about S.D. psychoprophylaxis we have conducted a study on the effect of this treatment on 9 patients, 5 bipolar and 4 unipolar depressives (Papadimitriou and collaborators, 1981). An outline of this study will be presented here.
The patients fulfilled the following criteria: 1) A diagnosis of primary affective disorder 2) Age below 65 years 3) Negative history for serious physical illness 4) A drug-free period of at least 15 days before initation òf treatment. The mean age of the patients was 40.55±11.01, there were 3 men and 6 women, duration of illness ranged from 1 to 25 years. One bipolar and all unipolar patients had received prophylactic treatment with lithium and tricyclic drugs respectively, without success. Three patients had attempted suicide in the past. With one exception all patients received one S.D. session per week.
Response to treatment was characterized as positive if the frequency of attacks decreased and the duration of normothymia increased after administration of P.S.D. in comparison to the same parameters before initiation of P.S.D.
Five patients (3 unipolar and 2 bipolar) responded to treatment, three patients (2 bipolar and one unipolar) failed to respond and in one patient the effect could not be evaluated.
With respect to the profile of the responder to prophylactic S.D. reliable conclusions would be impossible to draw due to the small sample studied. Our preliminary observations indicate that the responder is probably a woman in her mid-30s with rapid-cycling depression and a positive family history for mental illness. Responders and non-responders were not differentiated significantly with respect to premorbid personality, age at onset of illness and marital status.
Response of "rapid cyclers" to prophylactic S.D. is of more than theoretical importance as these patients don't seem to benefit from lithium. It is interesting to note that both patients of Kjellman, Larsson and Thorell (1977) were also "rapid cyclers".
Thus, if our own and the Scandinavian group's observations are confirmed by further research, then prophylactic S.D. might be considered as the method of choice for prophylactic management of patients with rapid cycling affective disorders.

ACKNOWLEDGEMENT
This work was partly supported by grant 88/1980 of Onassion Foundation.

REFERENCES

Bhanji, S., and G.A. Roy (1975). Br. J. Psychiat., 127, 222-226.
Bhanji, S., G.A. Roy and C. Baulieu (1978). Acta Psychiat. Scand., 58, 379-383.
Boston collaborative drug surveillance program: Adverse reaction to the tricyclic antidepressant drugs (1972). Lancet, i, 529-531.
Christodoulou, G.N., D.E. Malliaras, E.P. Lykouras, G.N. Papadimitriou, and C.N. Stefanis (1978a). Am. J. Psychiatry, 135, 375-376.
Christodoulou, G.N., E.P. Lykouras, G.N. Papadimitriou, D.E. Malliaras, and C.N. Stefanis (1978b). Possible prophylactic effect of sleep deprivation in recurrent affective disorders. 2nd World Congress of Biological Psychiatry, Barcelona.
Coull, D.C., J. Crooks, I. Dingwall-Fordyce, A.M. Scott, and R.D. Weir (1971). Lancet, ii, 590-591.
Dunner, D.L., and B.R. Fieve (1974). Arch. Gen. Psychiat., 30, 229-233.
Gerner, R.H., R.M. Post, J. Christian-Gillin, and W.E. Bunney Jr. (1978). J. Psychiat. Res., 15, 21-40.
Imlah, N.W., E. Ryan, and J.A. Harrington (1965). J. Neuropsychopharm., 4, 439-442.
Kjellman, B.F., M. Larsson, and L.H. Thorell (1977). Prophylactic sleep deprivation therapy. A pilot study. 7th World Congress of Psychiatry, Honolulu.
Larsen, J.K., M.L. Lingberg, and B. Skovgaard (1976). Acta Psychiat. Scand., 54, 167-173.
Mindham, R.H.S. (1981). Continuation therapy with tricyclic antidepressants in relapsing depressive illness. In G.N. Christodoulou, editor, Aspects of Preventive Psychiatry, Karger, Basel (in press).
Papadimitriou, G.N., G.N. Christodoulou, G.M. Trikkas, D.E. Malliaras, E.P. Lykouras, and C.N. Stefanis (1981). Sleep deprivation psychoprophylaxis in recurrent affective disorders. In G.N. Christodoulou, editor. Aspects of Preventive Psychiatry, Karger, Basel (in press).
Pflug , B., and R. Tölle (1971). Int. J. Pharmacopsychiat., 6, 187-196.
Prien, R.F., C.J. Klett, and E.M. Caffey Jr. (1973). Arch. Gen. Psychiat., 25, 420-425.
Roy, A., and S. Bhanji (1976). Postgrad. Med. J., 52, 50-52.
Schilgen, B., and R. Tölle (1980) Arch. Gen. Psychiat., 37, 267-271.
Seager, C.P., and R.L. Bird (1962). J. Ment. Sci., 108, 704-707.
Stevenson, G., and J. Geoghegan (1951). Am. J. Psychiatry, 107, 743
Van Praag, H.M., and S. de Haan (1980). 5-HTP and lithium prophylaxis in uni- and bipolar depression. Report 536. Abstracts of the 12th CINP Congress, supplement to: Progress in Neuropsychopharmacology, Pergamon Press, Oxford.
Vogel, G.W., F. Vogel, R.S. Mc Abee, and A.J. Thurmond (1980). Arch. Gen. Psychiat. 37, 247-253.